Hearing Science
FUNDAMENTALS

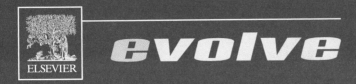

∴ *To access your Instructor and Student Resources, visit:*

http://evolve.elsevier.com/Lass/hearing

Evolve® Instructor Resources for *Lass: Hearing Science Fundamentals,* **First Edition,** offer the following features:

Instructor Resources

- **Test Bank**
- **Course Syllabus**
- **Image Collection**

Student and Instructor Resources

- **Archie Animations**
- **Word-Building Exercises**
- **Practice Test Questions**
- **Anatomy Labeling Exercises**

Hearing Science
FUNDAMENTALS

Norman J. Lass, PhD
Professor of Speech Pathology and Audiology
West Virginia University
Morgantown, WV

Charles M. Woodford, PhD
Professor Emeritus of Speech Pathology and Audiology
West Virginia University
Morgantown, WV

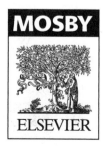

MOSBY

ELSEVIER

11830 Westline Industrial Drive
St. Louis, Missouri 63146

HEARING SCIENCE FUNDAMENTALS

ISBN-13: 978-0-323-04342-7
ISBN-10: 0-323-04342-9

Library of Congress Control Number: 2006941029

Publishing Director: Linda Duncan
Editor: Kathryn Falk
Associate Developmental Editor: Andrew Grow
Publishing Services Manager: Patricia Tannian
Senior Project Manager: Anne Altepeter
Cover Designer: Paula Ruckenbrod
Text Designer: Paula Ruckenbrod

Printed in the United States of America

Last digit is the print number: 9 8 7 6 5 4 3 2 1

PREFACE

Hearing Science Fundamentals addresses basic concepts in hearing science in an understandable manner to facilitate the learning of technical material by both undergraduate and graduate students. The book contains numerous student-friendly features, including the following:

- Learning objectives and key terms at the beginning of each chapter to prepare the student for learning the chapter contents
- More than 80 clear, two-color anatomical and line illustrations to help in understanding important, technical concepts
- Key terms defined in the margin notes throughout the text to reinforce learning
- Question-and-answer boxes to reinforce important information presented in the text
- Study questions at the end of each chapter for review of chapter contents
- Suggested readings at the end of each chapter for further clarification and study of the technical contents of each chapter
- A glossary of important terms used throughout the text (terms included in the glossary are in boldface type the first time they appear in the text) to enhance learning for students
- Exercises for each chapter provided at the end of the book can be used for self-study or for graded assignments
- A website for instructors containing a 200-question test bank, sample course syllabi, and an image collection of figures from the text. For students, animations, word-building exercises, practice test questions, and anatomy labeling exercises are included on the website.

These features make *Hearing Science Fundamentals* useful not only to students in facilitating the learning process but also to instructors for explaining technical concepts; providing a source of questions and illustrations for quizzes, examinations, and in-class learning exercises; and assigning additional readings on selected topics.

The book contains nine chapters that are divided into four sections: *Acoustics, Structure and Function, Psychoacoustics, and Pathologies.* The first section, *Acoustics*, contains one chapter: **Basic Acoustics.** This chapter introduces students to important concepts associated with sound, including conditions necessary to create sound, properties of vibrating systems, sinusoidal (simple harmonic) motion, sine curves and their spatial (amplitude and wavelength) as well as temporal (period, frequency, phase, and velocity) features, and characteristics of complex sounds. Also included is a discussion of sound propagation and interference as well as the phenomenon of resonance, specifically cavity (acoustical) resonance involving the tube model, which has direct relevance to hearing because of its analogy to the human external auditory canal. Finally, this chapter addresses the concept of the decibel. An understanding of these concepts will assist readers in applying basic concepts in acoustics to an understanding of the hearing process.

The second section, *Structure and Function*, contains three chapters intended to teach students the basic anatomy and physiology of the auditory mechanism. Chapter 2, **Anatomy and Physiology of the Conductive Auditory Mechanism,** describes the structures involved in conducting vibrational sound energy from outside the head through the outer ear (auricle and external auditory canal), tympanic membrane, and middle ear (ossicular chain) to the inner ear. Also included is a detailed description of the nonacoustic functions of the conductive mechanism (the role of ceruminous and sebaceous glands and curvature of the ear canal in protecting the tympanic membrane) as well as its acoustic function, including the resonance of the external auditory canal and the conversion of acoustic energy from the auricle and external auditory canal to mechanical energy at the tympanic membrane and through the ossicular chain of the middle ear. The transformer action function of the middle ear is discussed, including the condensation effect, lever action of the malleus and incus, and curved membrane buckling mechanism of the tympanic membrane. Finally, the function of the auditory (eustachian) tube and the two middle ear muscles (tensor tympani and stapedius) are presented.

Chapter 3, **Anatomy and Physiology of the Sensory Mechanism,** is concerned with the auditory portion of the inner ear contained in the cochlea, a very complex structure about whose function much is still unknown. All information that is necessary to understand speech, interpret sounds indicating danger to the organism, or appreciate music must be coded in this tiny structure, which is approximately 35 mm long. The anatomical structure of the cochlea is described, including its three canals and the organ of Corti, which resides in one of the canals. In addition, the outer and inner hair cells of the organ of Corti and their function are addressed. The function of the cochlea is very complex and not fully understood. Mechanical, electrochemical, and active processes contribute to the conversion from mechanical movement of parts of the conductive mechanism (tympanic membrane and ossicular chain) to the neural code that allows us to detect and interpret acoustic aspects of our environment. The mechanical properties and active processes involved in the sensory mechanism as well as cochlear electrophysiology and single-cell electrical activity are described.

A comprehensive description of the anatomical structure and physiological function of the central auditory mechanism, including the afferent and efferent central auditory pathways, is presented in Chapter 4, **Anatomy and Physiology of the Central Auditory Mechanism.** The central auditory system is much more than a conduit from the cochlea to the brain. While actions like the startle reflex, acoustic reflex, and localization responses are initiated at levels that are peripheral to the cerebral cortex, complex analysis of speech, music, and multisensory construction of our environment take place within the cortex. Thus, complexity of function usually increases from the eighth cranial nerve to the cerebral cortex. In addition to information transmission from the cochlea to higher centers, there is also neural energy flow, much of which is inhibitory or suppressive, from higher centers to lower areas, including the cochlea. Although the function of the central auditory system is not completely understood, much is learned from instances in which its function is impaired, such as from cerebrovascular accidents, head trauma, and (central) auditory processing disorders.

The third section of the book, *Psychoacoustics,* contains four chapters about how sound is perceived through the auditory pathway. In Chapter 5, **Normal Hearing,** several aspects of auditory sensitivity are addressed, including the frequency, intensity, and duration of the auditory stimulus, mode of stimulus presentation, psychophysical methods, and listener characteristics such as preparatory set and age. The concept of "normal hearing" is discussed, and it is concluded that hearing sensitivity is dynamic, with the quantification of threshold partially depending on the operational definition of the examiner. Clinical assessment of auditory sensitivity, the primary cues (intensity and time) associated with localization of sound sources, and hearing by bone conduction are also addressed. It is concluded that the processes involved in normal hearing are not simple. The role assumed by the auditory and other sensory systems is very complex, and this complexity and subtlety of interaction is usually taken for granted as long as the systems function as intended.

Chapter 6, **Masking,** addresses the concept of masking, a process in which the threshold of one sound (the signal) is raised by the simultaneous presentation of another sound (the masker). Masking involves the introduction of a sound (the masker) to an ear to preclude a person from hearing another sound (the signal) in the same ear. This chapter includes the masking of tones by other tones, masking as a function of noise level, the concept and importance of the critical band in masking, wideband noise as a masker of pure tones, temporal (forward and backward) masking, and masking level difference. Also discussed is masking in clinical audiology, including the concepts of cross-hearing, cross-skull attenuation, crossover, speech (or pink) noise, and effective masking.

Chapter 7, **Loudness and Pitch,** addresses the measurement of these subjective perceptions of the objective physical attributes of intensity and frequency, respectively. It is concluded that both loudness and pitch are very complex psychophysical phenomena. Although it is possible to scale both loudness (in phons and sones) and pitch (in mels) with very high intra-subject consistency, there are components of each that are not fully understood. Neither loudness nor pitch varies directly with their physical counterparts of intensity and frequency, respectively, while each is influenced primarily by those physical properties.

Chapter 8, **Differential Sensitivity,** is concerned with how much of a change in a physical parameter of an auditory signal must be made before it is noticed by a listener. This minimum change that is necessary for the signal to be detected is called a *just noticeable difference* (jnd) or *difference limen.* The Fechner/Weber law is discussed, and some findings pertaining to difference thresholds for the acoustic parameters of intensity, frequency, and time are presented. Although there is variability in findings across subjects, methods, and studies, and while there are significant differences between empirically derived data and results predicted by Fechner/Weber's law, there is also much agreement between them. The general principle that the magnitude of change necessary for detection of a signal increases with the magnitude of the standard (fixed) stimulus applies over a broad range of stimulus parameters in all sensory systems.

The fourth and final section of the book, *Pathologies,* is covered in Chapter 9, **Pathologies of the Auditory Mechanism.** This chapter addresses primarily pathologies that affect the outer ear, middle ear, and inner ear. Outer ear pathologies include agenesis (absence) of the auricle, aplasia (deformation) of the auricle, frostbitten auricle, and disfigurement of the auricle, called *cauliflower ear.* These pathologies present a cosmetic and, in some cases, a health problem. Other outer ear pathologies that can potentially cause a conductive type of hearing loss include a stenosis (narrowing) and congenital atresia (complete closure) of the external auditory canal, external otitis (swimmer's ear), and impacted cerumen. Middle ear pathologies include eustachian tube dysfunction, otitis media, otosclerosis, ossicular discontinuity, and cholesteatoma. Among the causes of inner ear pathologies are noise exposure, ototoxic drugs, viral infections, Meniere's disease, and presbycusis/socioacusis. Finally, disorders of the central auditory mechanism are discussed.

It was our intention to write a basic, understandable text for use in classes that is appropriate for undergraduate and graduate students who are being exposed for the first time to hearing science, thereby facilitating their learning of technical material in basic acoustics, anatomy and physiology of the auditory mechanism, and psychoacoustics. We have brought our combined 60+ years of higher education teaching experience and understanding of the learning process to the writing of this book, which is the result of a compilation of material used in classes for a number of years. The contents of this volume will not only provide readers with an understanding of important basic concepts but also will make them aware of current unresolved issues in hearing science that will facilitate a deeper appreciation for the complex processes involved in audition.

Norman J. Lass
Charles M. Woodford

ACKNOWLEDGMENTS

We acknowledge our former mentors who provided us not only with an understanding of and appreciation for the complexity of the hearing and speech mechanisms but also, more importantly, with the scholarly models for us to emulate. They informed us and inspired us by their own scholarliness and dedication. In particular, we owe a debt of gratitude to professors J. Douglas Noll, Kenneth W. Burk, Ralph L. Shelton, John F. Michel, Donald Henderson, Herbert Wright, and Charles Marean. The commitment of these individuals to their teaching and research has had a profound influence on our education and subsequent professional careers. We will always be indebted to them.

We also acknowledge the very helpful comments and suggestions offered by Laurie Sparks of Elsevier in her review of our writing as well as her assistance in the preparation of the glossary and chapter study questions. Her input has been crucial to the completion of the text. We also are indebted to Kathy Falk, acquisitions editor, and Andrew Grow, associate developmental editor at Elsevier. Their suggestions, comments, reminders, perseverance, and never-ending patience and assistance have allowed us to bring this writing project to completion. The work of Anne Altepeter, senior project manager at Elsevier, is also acknowledged. Without her assistance, the book would never have been published in a timely manner. It was a pleasure to work with the staff at Elsevier because of their competence, caring, and professionalism.

Finally, to our wives, Martha and Robin, whose never-ending patience and understanding were most helpful to us throughout the duration of this writing project, our deepest gratitude and appreciation.

Norman J. Lass
Charles M. Woodford

CONTENTS

ACOUSTICS

Basic Acoustics

KEY TERMS

Sound
Molecules
Mass
Elasticity
Spring-mass model
Inertia
Resistance
Sinusoidal motion (simple harmonic motion)
Pure tone
Compression (condensation)
Rarefaction (expansion)
J.B. Fourier
Fourier analysis
Amplitude
Peak amplitude
Peak-to-peak amplitude
Root mean square (rms)
Wavelength
Cycle
Period
Frequency
Pitch
Phase
Velocity
Reverberations
Waveform
Spectrum
Complex sounds
Periodicity
Aperiodicity
Noise
Fundamental
Harmonics
Wide-band noise
Spectral envelope
Impedance
Stiffness
Resistance
Transduction
Resonant frequency (natural frequency)
Sounding board resonance (sounding board effect)
Damping

SIDE NOTES

Rest position
Frequency response curve (resonance curve)
Bandwidth
Physicists' zero
Decibel
Logarithm
Sound pressure level (SPL)
Hearing level (HL)
Hearing threshold level (HTL)

LEARNING OBJECTIVES

After studying this chapter, the student will be able to do the following:

1. Define sound and identify the elements necessary for the production of sound.
2. Describe the motion of a sine wave.
3. Describe the two spatial and five temporal concepts associated with sine waves.
4. Describe the relationships between frequency/period and frequency/wavelength.
5. Describe the difference between simple and complex sounds.
6. Differentiate periodicity and aperiodicity in sounds.
7. Define fundamental and harmonics of complex sounds.
8. Define harmonics in terms of energy distribution on a discrete (line) spectrum.
9. Identify the three components of impedance and explain how each affects energy transfer.
10. Calculate the resonant frequencies of an inanimate tube system and describe their relevance to hearing.
11. Discuss the importance of the decibel, how it is computed, and how it is used in describing the energy of a sound.
12. Define the following concepts:
    a. frequency response curve
    b. undamped resonators
    c. damped resonators
    d. bandwidth

This chapter addresses basic concepts associated with sound. Its purpose is to help the reader gain insight into basic acoustics, which can then be applied to an understanding of the processing of auditory signals, both simple (e.g., pure tones) and complex (e.g., speech sounds).

Aspects of sound presented here include basic parameters, spatial and temporal aspects, spectral and pressure measurements, and sound propagation and conduction. This chapter is not intended to be a comprehensive coverage of acoustics, but rather an introduction to those aspects of sound that are most important in understanding the coupling of our external acoustic environment to our perceptual mechanism through the auditory system.

SOUND

Sound can be defined as *a condition of disturbance of particles in a medium.* Three components are necessary for the production of sound: (1) an energy source, (2) a body capable of vibration, and (3) a transmitting medium. The propagating medium of most relevance for us is *air.* If a portion of the medium of air could be observed microscopically, it would be found to consist of billions of air particles called **molecules.** A further discovery would be that these molecules are consistently spaced with respect to one another.

The properties common to the medium of air and other media used for the transmission of sound waves are mass, elasticity, and inertia. Mass is any form of matter (solid, liquid, gas). The particles in a medium such as air consist of mass. If a medium has **elasticity,** it is able to resist permanent distortion to its original shape or the distribution of its molecules. Thus, it possesses the property of *springiness,* or a propensity to return to its original position when the forces of displacement are removed. This elasticity resulting in springiness is also referred to as *stiffness.* Because air is not observable, it is difficult to think of it in terms of having a shape that can be distorted. A visual aid useful for an understanding of these concepts is the **spring-mass model** (Figure 1-1).

In Figure 1-1, the initial portion *(A)* depicts a weight attached to a spring on a trapdoor. The spring is attached to a solid suspension system. Note that the spring is in a neutral position, neither extended nor compressed. The second portion *(B)* shows the effects of opening the trapdoor, at which point the force of gravity moves the weight downward until the elasticity of the spring overcomes the effect of gravitational force on the mass. The movement then changes to an upward motion. This up-and-down motion will continue until the resistance of the air results in the cessation of motion. This phenomenon can be

▼ **SIDE NOTES**

▼ **Sound** a condition of disturbance of particles in a medium.

▼ **Mass** Any form of matter.

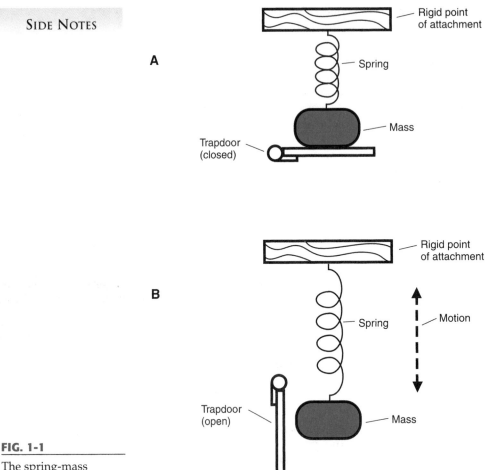

FIG. 1-1

The spring-mass
model.

▼ **Inertia** Principle stating
that a body in motion
tends to remain in motion,
whereas a body at rest
tends to remain at rest.

readily demonstrated by attaching a small weight to a rubber band.
Using gravity as the force, drop the weight, and observe the elasticity of
the rubber band and the mass of the weight interact in an up-and-down
motion.

If we vary the size of the weight and the elasticity of the rubber band,
we can observe the differences in movement related to the various combinations. The molecules (mass) in air behave as if they had springs
attached to them (springiness = elasticity), which allows them to be
moved from and returned to their original rest position. Because of
inertia, however, they do not stop. **Inertia** is a property common to all
matter: a body in motion tends to remain in motion, whereas a body at
rest tends to remain at rest (unless acted on by an external force). Because
the molecules are in motion as they move toward their rest position, they
will not stop at this position, but rather will continue to move beyond it.

An energy source is used to activate a vibrator of some kind; the energy source required often depends on the vibrator itself. A vibrator such as a tuning fork needs to be struck against a hard surface in order for it to be activated. Drum heads need to be hit with a stick or mallet to cause disturbances in the medium. If air is forced between tightly constricted lips, a buzzing sound can be made, which is used as a sound source for trumpet and tuba players. Air is also the primary propagating medium for speech production.

A vibrating body will not remain in motion indefinitely because of another basic physical property: **resistance.** Whereas mass and stiffness store energy within a system, resistance dissipates energy. This dissipation occurs primarily by *transduction* (conversion) into thermal energy. In a mechanical system, mass, stiffness, and resistance constitute *impedance,* which represents overall opposition to energy transfer. The dissipation of vibratory energy is referred to as *damping.*

Pressure is force distributed over a particular area. In discussing pressure, originally both the applied force and the area over which it was distributed were noted, that is, dyne/cm², with the *dyne* being a measure of force and square centimeters (cm²) a measure of area. More recently, pressure is measured in units of *pascals* (Pa), in honor of Blaise Pascal, a seventeenth-century mathematician. For example, 0.0002 dyne/cm² is equal to 20 micropascals (μPa).

Thus, when variations in pressure from current atmospheric pressure occur with a frequency of occurrence that is detectable by the auditory system, sound is produced. For this to happen, it is necessary to have something cause pressure to vary, usually an object capable of vibrating, some source of energy to cause this object to vibrate, and some medium to transport the pressure variations caused by the vibrating object to our ears.

SIDE NOTES

▼ **Resistance** Dissipation of energy, primarily by transduction (conversion) to heat.

Sinusoidal Motion

Describing sound in such a way as to visualize it is not a straightforward process because of the abstract nature of the concept of sound. One way is by discussing the simplest type of sound wave motion that can occur in a medium. This simple wave motion is called **sinusoidal motion** (or **simple harmonic motion**). Sinusoidal motion is a disturbance in a medium that occurs when devices such as tuning forks and clock pendulums are activated. Figure 1-2 illustrates sinusoidal motion as it is being traced from the movements of a clock pendulum.

If a sheet of paper could be pulled underneath the back-and-forth movements (*oscillations*) of a swinging pendulum with a pen attached to the bottom of the pendulum, the picture of a sine wave would emerge on the paper. The pendulum would begin its movement from a point of

▼ **Sinusoidal motion** A disturbance in a medium in which particles are displaced perpendicular to the direction of the disturbance.

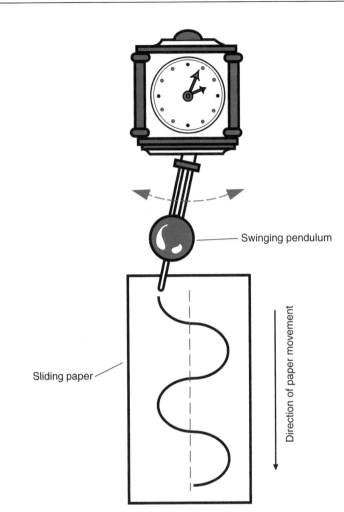

Swinging pendulum

Sliding paper

Direction of paper movement

FIG.1-2

Sinusoidal motion.

rest, move in one direction to a point of maximum displacement, return to its point of rest, go through its point of rest to maximum displacement in the opposite direction, and then again return to its rest position. The result is a *sine wave tracing,* which is a graph displaying two basic properties of motion: time and displacement.

The sound that is generated from vibrators that produce sinusoidal movement is often designated as a pure tone, a sound that has almost all its energy located at one frequency. Pure tones are rarely heard in everyday situations; most of the sounds that we routinely hear in our environment are *complex* in that their energy is concentrated at more than a single frequency.

When sinusoidal wave motion disturbs the particles of the medium, they react in a predictable way. As the pendulum or tuning fork tine

▼ **Pure tone** A sound that has almost all its energy located in a single frequency.

begins to move from rest to maximum displacement in one direction, the particles in the medium are pushed closer toward each other; they are said to be in a state of **compression** (or **condensation**). Maximum compression takes place at the point of maximum excursion of the vibrating pendulum or tuning fork tine. As the pendulum or tuning fork tine begins to move in the opposite direction, the particles attempt to return to their original positions (because of elasticity), but they overshoot that position (because of inertia) before coming to rest again. This overshoot, where the particles are spread apart more than they normally would be, is called a state of **rarefaction** (or **expansion**).

These condensations and rarefactions are the actual sound disturbances that travel through the medium from the sound source. It should be noted that the particles (molecules) themselves are not moving through the medium. The particles near an environmental noise during sound production will move around their points of origin *(rest positions)*, but once the sound disturbance has traveled away from the point of origin, those particles will return to their rest positions. Thus, the disturbance will have moved away from the noise source, but not the individual particles in the medium; they will simply be displaced temporarily from their rest position.

The sine wave tracing can provide a spatial or a temporal picture of particle disturbances in the medium. As a *spatial* picture, the sine wave tracing indicates the relative positions of the particles in the medium at a single instant in time. As a *temporal* picture, it can be used to study the movement of a single particle over time as it changes its location around its rest position. Each view of the sine wave tracing has a set of terms associated with it.

J.B. Fourier, a French mathematician who lived in the early nineteenth century, showed that any complex periodic sound wave disturbance can be mathematically broken down into its individual sine wave (*pure tone* or *sinusoidal*) components, which vary in terms of frequency, amplitude, and phase relations with respect to one another. This mathematical analysis of complex signals into their sinusoidal components is called **Fourier analysis.** Thus, when we look at a pure tone, we are studying the most basic component of sound.

Spatial Concepts

Amplitude

Amplitude refers to the maximum displacement of the particles of a medium. It is related perceptually to the magnitude (loudness) of the sound. Amplitude indicates the energy (intensity) of a sound; it is usually measured from the baseline (point of rest) to the point of maximum dis-

▼ **Amplitude** Maximum displacement of the particles of a medium.

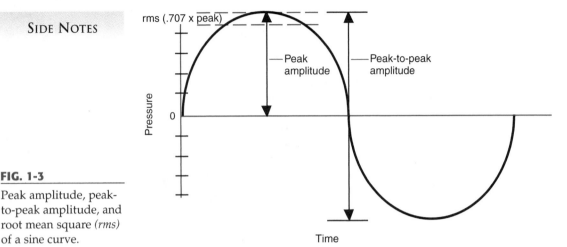

FIG. 1-3

Peak amplitude, peak-to-peak amplitude, and root mean square (*rms*) of a sine curve.

placement on the wave form (Figure 1-3). This linear measurement is called **peak amplitude** measurement.

The distance between the baseline and the point of maximum displacement is related to the movement of the swinging pendulum or tuning fork tine as it moves from rest to maximum excursion in one direction. In other words, amplitude is related to the point of maximum displacement of a particular vibrating object. In the case of the spring-mass model, it represents maximum excursion of the mass from its rest position (Figure 1-4). Note that maximum displacement occurs at the peaks of the sine wave (points 2 and 4) in Figure 1-4.

In some instances, amplitude measurements are made on the sine wave tracings from the point of maximum displacement in one direction to the point of maximum displacement in the other direction, instead of from baseline to the point of maximum displacement in one direction. This linear measurement is called **peak-to-peak amplitude** measurement (see Figure 1-3). It is important to indicate whether the amplitude being reported is in terms of "peak" or "peak-to-peak" measurements.

Measurement of amplitude of sound pressure is often a **root mean square (rms)** value, which is mathematically the square root of the average of all instantaneous variations of pressure squared within the sine wave. This value, in a sinusoid, is equivalent to 0.707 times the peak value and represents the average sound pressure variations within the sinusoid (see Figure 1-3).

Amplitude is related to the measurement of intensity at rms, which can be expressed in terms of sound pressure level or power. The *decibel* (dB) is the most common unit used to express sound intensity when amplitude is being measured in terms of sound pressure or power (see later discussion).

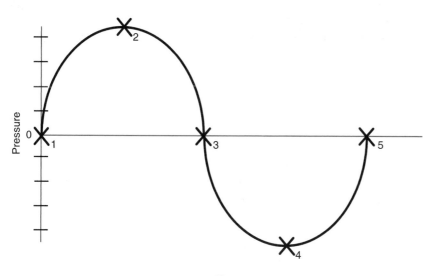

1, 3, 5 = zero displacement
1, 3, 5 = zero pressure
2, 4 = maximum displacement
2, 4 = maximum pressure

FIG. 1-4

Particle displacement and pressure.

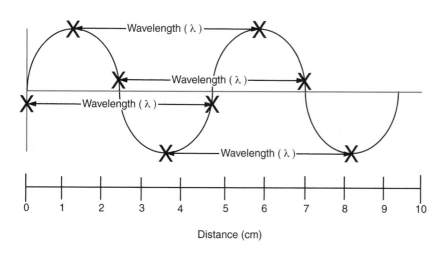

FIG. 1-5

Wavelength (λ).

Wavelength

Wavelength (λ), another spatial term, is a linear measurement that refers to the distance that a sound wave disturbance can travel during one complete cycle of vibration. More specifically, wavelength can be defined as the distance between points of identical phase in two adjacent cycles of a wave (Figure 1-5). Wavelength can be expressed in feet, meters, or

▼ **Wavelength** Distance that a sound wave disturbance travels during one complete cycle of vibration.

centimeters and, as discussed later, it is inversely related to the frequency of the sound being produced. Phase is described in the following section.

Temporal Concepts

Cycle

Cycle is a time concept referring to vibrator movement from rest position to maximum displacement in one direction, back to rest, to maximum displacement in the opposite direction, and back to rest again (Figure 1-6).

Period

▼ **Period** Time needed for a vibrator to complete one complete cycle of vibration.

Period is the time (usually expressed in milliseconds; 1 msec is $\frac{1}{1000}$ of a second) that it takes for a vibrator to complete one complete cycle of vibration (Figure 1-7). The period of the sine curve in Figure 1-7 is 1 msec because it took that amount of time to complete one cycle of vibration.

Frequency

▼ **Frequency** Number of complete cycles occurring during a certain time period, usually 1 second.

Frequency is the number of complete cycles that occur during a certain time period, usually 1 second (Figure 1-8). Frequency is expressed in *cycles per second* (cps) or *hertz* (Hz) (in honor of Heinrich Hertz, the first person to demonstrate electromagnetic waves) or, more often, in kilohertz (1 kHz = 1000 Hz). In Figure 1-8 the sine curve has two complete cycles of vibration in 1 msec; therefore, its frequency is 2000 cps (or Hz) (2/0.001 = 2000). That is, two cycles in 1 msec ($\frac{1}{1000}$ of a second) results in a period of 0.5 msec (1 msec = 0.001 second). If the swinging pen-

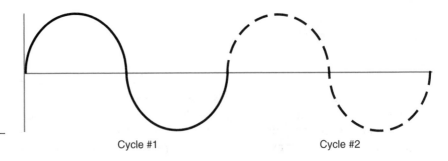

FIG. 1-6

Cycles of a sine curve.

Cycle #1   Cycle #2

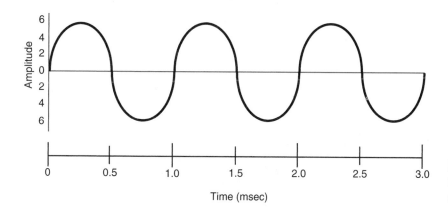

FIG. 1-7

Period of a 1000-Hz sine wave.

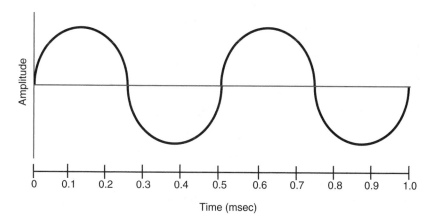

FIG. 1-8

Frequency of a sine wave.

dulum or tuning fork tine or mass in the spring-mass model completes 100 cycles in 1 second, then its frequency of vibration is 100 cps (Hz) and its period is 10 msec ($\frac{1}{100} = 0.01$ sec $\times 1000 = 10$ msec).

The **pitch** of a signal is the perceptual correlate of frequency. For example, a 100-Hz pure tone would be perceived as being lower in pitch than a 1000-Hz pure tone. As is true for loudness, pitch determination requires human perceptual judgments of the sound.

Phase

Phase represents the point in the cycle at which the vibrator is located at a given instant in time. If we were to transpose the two portions of the sine wave so that the top and bottom portions joined, forming a circle or ellipse, it becomes evident that any portion of that figure can be defined in degrees of a circle. The result of this notation is shown in Figure 1-9. Two sinusoids are *in phase* when their wave disturbances crest and trough at the same time (Figure 1-9, *A*) and *out of phase* when they do not

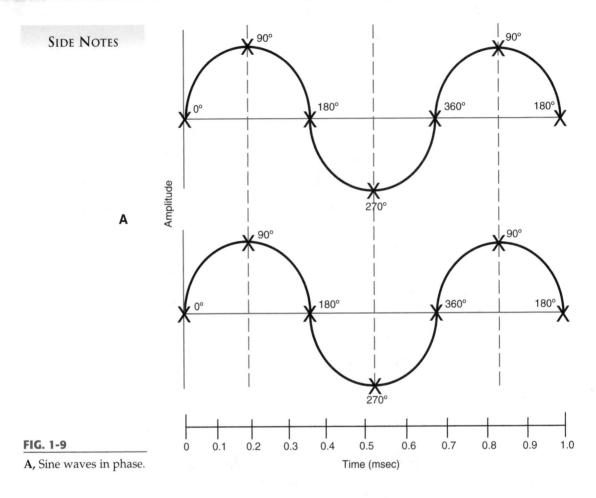

A

Amplitude

0°   90°   180°   270°   360°   180°

0   0.1   0.2   0.3   0.4   0.5   0.6   0.7   0.8   0.9   1.0

Time (msec)

FIG. 1-9

A, Sine waves in phase.

(Figure 1-9, *B*). Given this description, the exact relationship of any sine waves may be defined as a certain number of degrees out of phase with each other. For example, Figure 1-9, *B,* shows two sine waves that are 180 degrees (180°) out of phase.

Velocity

▼ **Velocity** Speed of sound through a transmitting medium.

Velocity is the speed of sound through a transmitting medium. The average speed of sound in the medium of air is approximately 1100 feet per second, or 340 meters per second, or 34,000 centimeters per second. Different sources will vary slightly with regard to these figures because there are some differences in the speed of sound in air, and velocity is measured at different heights above sea level and at different temperatures. The speed of sound in air is relatively constant because of

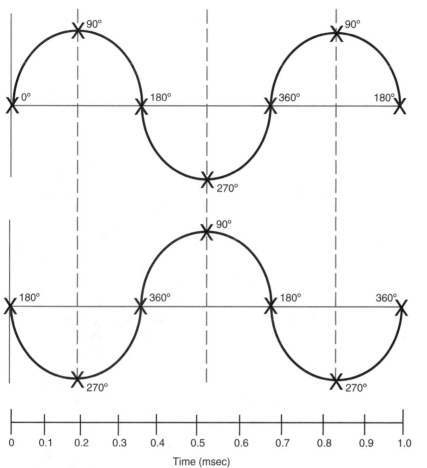

B

FIG. 1-9, cont'd
B, Sine waves out of phase.

the elastic and inertial properties of a given medium. Water has different elastic and inertial properties than air, and consequently the speed of sound is faster in water than in air.

Q & A

Question:
Why do sound waves travel faster through the medium of steel than through the medium of air?

Answer:
Although the density of steel (a solid) is greater than that of air (a gas), the elasticity of steel is also greater than that of air, and elasticity is the primary factor in determining the velocity of sound waves.

Frequency/Period Relationship

An inverse relationship exists between period and frequency. This reciprocal relationship is expressed in the following formula:

$$Frequency = 1/Period$$

If the frequency for a particular sound wave is 1000 Hz, its period would be 0.001 second (period = $\frac{1}{1000}$ second). Because *period* is the time needed for the completion of one cycle of vibration, as frequency is increased (more cycles per second), period will be reduced (less time for the completion of any one particular cycle). Thus, as frequency is increased, period decreases proportionately (Figure 1-10). For example, a pure tone of 250 Hz will have a longer period $\frac{1}{250}$ or 4 msec, or 0.0045 sec) than one of 1000 Hz ($\frac{1}{1000}$ or 1 msec, or 0.001 sec).

Frequency/Wavelength Relationship

An inverse relationship exists between the time concept of frequency and the spatial concept of wavelength. As frequency is increased, wavelength becomes shorter, and as frequency is decreased, wavelength becomes longer. Because the number of cycles is increased within the same unit of time, each cycle will take less time and cover a shorter distance (see Figure 1-10). It is an established fact in environmental acoustics that lower frequencies are more difficult to absorb than higher frequencies because of their longer wavelengths. A frequency of 100 Hz, for example, has a wavelength of approximately 11 feet, whereas a frequency of 10,000 Hz has a wavelength of only approximately 1.2 inches. The 10,000-Hz tone could be absorbed by acoustical ceiling tile that is only a few inches thick. However, the 100-Hz frequency would require an unusually thick wall or some other type of acoustical treatment for it to be completely absorbed.

The relationship between frequency and wavelength can be expressed in the following formulas:

$$\lambda = v/f$$
$$f = v/\lambda$$

where f = frequency, λ = wavelength, and v = velocity (a constant; refers to the speed of sound).

Example 1: If the frequency of vibration for a particular sound wave disturbance is 100 Hz, the wavelength for that frequency would be 11.0 feet, or 3.4 meters, or 34,000 centimeters (wavelength = velocity/ frequency: 1100 feet per sec/100 Hz = 11.0 feet; or 340 meters per sec/100 Hz = 3.4 meters; or 34,000 cm per sec/100 Hz = 340 cm).

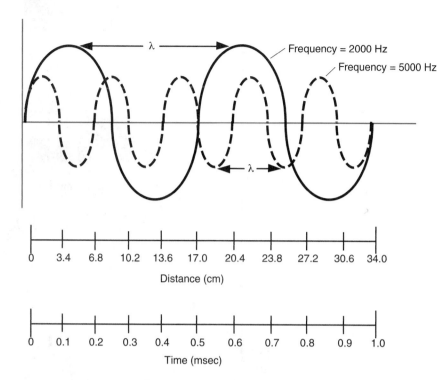

Frequency = 2000 Hz
Frequency = 5000 Hz

Distance (cm)

Time (msec)

SIDE NOTES

FIG. 1-10

Reciprocal relationship between frequency and period as well as frequency and wavelength.

In Example 1, if the unit of measurement for velocity is feet per second, the wavelength is expressed in feet. If the unit of measurement is meters per second, the wavelength is expressed in meters. It is important to note that the answer is not expressed in feet or meters *per second*, but in feet or meters. Wavelength is a linear measurement of the *distance* covered by a sound wave disturbance during one cycle of its vibration.

> *Example 2: If the wavelength for a particular sound wave disturbance is 1.1 feet, or 0.34 meter, the frequency for that sound wave disturbance would be 1000 Hz (frequency = velocity/wavelength: 1100 feet per sec/1.1 feet = 1000 Hz; or 340 meters per sec/0.34 meter = 1000 Hz).*

Sound Propagation and Interference

Once a sound wave strikes an object, three things can happen to it (Figure 1-11). First, the sound can simply continue as though the object were not there. The intervening object does nothing to impede the magnitude of the sound as it moves outward from the sound source. In this case an object (e.g., a wall) has been struck, but the sound disturbance keeps on going as though the object did not exist. Second, the sound energy being emitted can be *absorbed* by the object that has been struck.

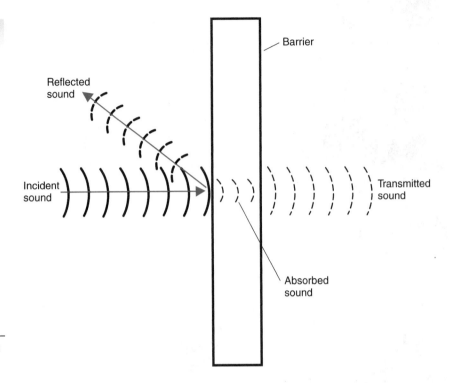

FIG. 1-11

Effects of sound waves striking an object.

▼ **Reverberations** Multiple or continuous reflected sounds that prolong the existence of a sound within a confined space.

If the object is a wall with absorptive properties, the sound energy enters the structure, is converted to thermal energy (heat), and is then dissipated. Third, when sound strikes an object, it can bounce off the object. When sound bounces off a wall, it is said to be *reflected*. If the reflections are multiple or continuous to the point where they actually prolong the existence of the sound within a confined space, they are referred to as reverberations, the prolongation of a sound through multiple or continuous reflections.

Complex Sounds

Thus far our discussion of basic acoustics has centered on simple sound disturbances. When sounds of varying frequency and intensity interact, the result may be displayed in a graph. An example of this graph appears in Figure 1-12, which shows the interaction of two pure tones of different frequency. These sinusoidal disturbances have been shown graphically on an amplitude-by-time display known as a **waveform** graph (Figure 1-12, *A*). Another method for displaying sound is to graph it in terms of amplitude as a function of frequency. When amplitude is plotted as a function of frequency, the resulting graph is referred to as a **spectrum** (Figure 1-12, *B*).

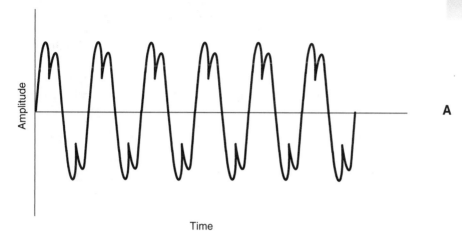

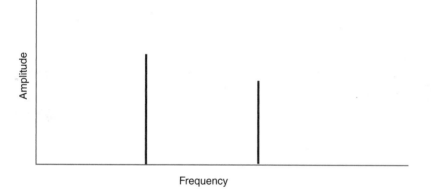

A

B

FIG. 1-12

A, Complex periodic waveform. **B,** Line spectrum.

The vertical length of the single line would be equal to the amplitude of the pure tone that has been graphed. A spectrum shows amplitude as a function of frequency at a single instant in time and has the advantage of allowing frequency to be read directly from the display. A waveform has the advantage of showing amplitude changes over time, but frequency would need to be calculated. The spectrum provides little advantage over the waveform display when viewing pure tones because all the energy is concentrated at a single frequency. However, when viewing complex sounds, in which there is energy at more than one frequency, the sound spectrum becomes more valuable.

Complex sounds differ from simple sounds in that they have energy distributed at more than one frequency. A single tuning fork generates a sound with energy concentrated at one frequency. If two tuning forks of different frequencies were activated simultaneously, the sound generated would consist of two frequencies and would therefore be considered complex in nature. The resultant waveform would no longer show smooth curves like that of the sine wave, and the spectrum would have two vertical lines, each line representing the frequency of vibration of one of the tuning forks vibrating simultaneously with the other (see Figure 1-12, *B*). Speech sounds, like the vowels of English, are very complex in that they have energy distributed at numerous frequencies, with amplitude variations at each of the frequencies involved. Figure 1-13 shows the sound spectrum for the vowel /i/ as in **beet**.

Periodicity vs. Aperiodicity

A periodic sound disturbance is one in which the wave shape repeats itself as a function of time; that is, the wave shape is said to have **periodicity** (see Figure 1-12, *A*). A pure tone that provides simple harmonic motion is, by definition, periodic, as is the swing of a pendulum or tuning fork tine. The pure tone has a clearly defined frequency because of the cyclical (periodic) behavior of the vibrator generating it.

An aperiodic sound disturbance is one in which the wave shape does not repeat itself as a function of time and therefore is said to have **aperiodicity**. Static on the radio and a sudden explosion are examples of an aperiodic sound disturbance. When these sounds are heard, they are usually perceived as **noise** because they lack any cyclical or repetitive

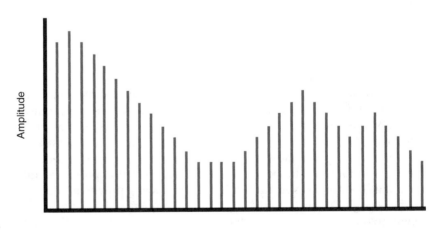

FIG. 1-13

Spectrum for /i/.

vibrations. Another, and perhaps more practical, definition of noise is *unwanted sound*; no matter how periodic your roommate's music is when you are studying, it may well fit within this psychological definition of *noise*.

Spectral displays of complex periodic and complex aperiodic sounds reveal the major differences between them. For complex periodic waves, the frequency of each component is a whole-number multiple of the component with the lowest frequency, called the **fundamental** (Figure 1-14). The first bar (i.e., the bar showing the lowest frequency) is the *fundamental frequency*, and the energy bars above it are whole-number multiples of the fundamental frequency, called **harmonics.** If the lowest bar of energy has a frequency of 100 Hz, the second energy bar would have a frequency of 200 Hz, the third would have a frequency of 300 Hz, and so on. The heights of the energy bars for the various frequencies in this spectrum refer to the relative amplitude for each pure tone making up this complex periodic sound. In this spectrum the pure-tone component with the highest concentration of energy (i.e., the greatest amplitude) is the *fundamental*, the component pure tone comprising this complex signal with the lowest frequency.

For complex aperiodic sounds, there is no fundamental frequency or harmonics because the disturbances produced do not set up any cyclical or repetitious behavior. Instead, energy is distributed throughout the sound spectrum at a particular instant in time. Figure 1-15, *A*, shows the spectrum for **wide-band noise**, which sounds like a prolonged "sh" sound. White noise has energy distributed evenly throughout the spectrum and is therefore effective for masking other sounds. Instead of having discrete lines (representing concentrations of energy or energy bars) like those used for complex periodic sound spectra, a graph/dis-

SIDE NOTES

▼ **Wide-band noise** Sound that has energy distributed evenly throughout the spectrum.

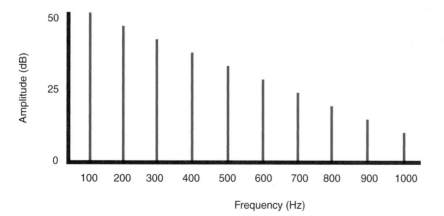

FIG. 1-14

Spectrum showing fundamental frequency and harmonics.

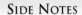
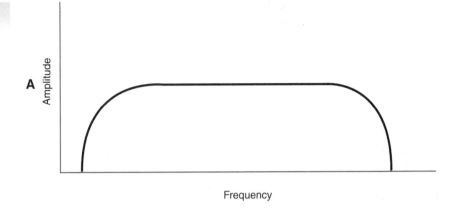

FIG. 1-15

A, Spectral envelope for white noise. **B,** Spectral envelope for /s/.

play called a **spectral envelope** is employed to show the distribution of energy for complex aperiodic sound disturbances.

The spectral envelope is a line running horizontally across the spectral graph which, in this case, because it is a flat line, indicates that energy is distributed evenly throughout the frequency range. If the spectrum is showing an aperiodic signal other than white noise, the spectral envelope would not be completely flat, but rather would show variations where higher or lower energy regions within the frequency range would be located. Figure 1-15, *B,* shows the spectrum for the speech sound /s/ (as in **s**un). In this instance there is a concentration of energy in the higher frequency range, and this concentration is shown by a "rise" in the spectral envelope for the frequencies where the energy concentration is located.

RESONANCE

Another way in which sound is modified after production is by a phenomenon called *resonance*. There are different types of resonance, but all are based on the same principles. As discussed earlier, impedance is defined as the overall opposition to flow of energy. This overall opposition consists of three components, which are mass, stiffness, and resistance in the systems discussed here. To define **mass,** it may be best to define *weight*, which is mass acted on by gravity. We may further appreciate mass with the question, "Which weighs more, a pound of feathers or a pound of lead?" The answer to this allegedly humorous question is that by definition the two weigh the same. However, if we envision a pound of feathers and a pound of lead, we see that the bulk in the two is very different; that is, because the mass of feathers is less than the mass of lead, it requires a larger volume of feathers to achieve 1 pound in weight.

Stiffness may be envisioned as "springiness" or elasticity. If we stretch a rubber band, the further we stretch it, the stiffer it becomes. Resistance in a mechanical system is afforded by friction. In a hydraulic system, resistance is increased as we adjust the nozzle on a garden hose, allowing a small stream of water to flow with a lot of pressure (force per unit area), as we increase resistance, or decreasing resistance so that water flows in a large volume with little pressure.

Mass and stiffness are energy-storing components of impedance, whereas **resistance** is an energy-dissipating component. We can appreciate this fact by thinking of rolling a lead ball up an incline. The larger the lead ball (the greater the mass), the more energy we must expend in getting it up the incline. When the ball is released, it rolls down the incline, expending the energy that we put into rolling it up. That is, it stored that energy. The moral of the story is that the more energy it takes to roll a ball up an incline, the more important it becomes to stay out of its way when it rolls down!

The energy storage aspect of stiffness becomes obvious if we think of compressing a spring or drawing a bow, as in bow and arrow. The more difficult it is to compress the spring or to draw the bow, the greater will be the reaction when either is released. The stiffness of the spring or bow has stored the energy put into compressing or drawing it.

Resistance changes the form of energy. We can neither create nor destroy energy; however, we can change its form, a process called transduction. On a cold day, we may rub our hands together to warm them. In doing this, the friction, or resistance, has changed some of the energy put into rubbing the hands together into heat energy. The mechanical energy then has been dissipated as heat, or transduced into heat energy.

▼ **Impedance**   Overall opposition to the flow of energy; consists of mass, stiffness, and resistance.

▼ **Transduction** The process of changing energy from one form to another.

Mass, stiffness, and resistance are all present in different proportions in every system that will be of interest to us. We will not talk about each in isolation, but rather in terms of which is proportionally greatest. It turns out that in any given system, the relative magnitude of the two energy-storing components of impedance (i.e., mass and stiffness) determines the rate at which a system will vibrate when set into vibration. Resistance will determine, other factors being constant, how long the system will vibrate. This can be demonstrated by taking a rubber band, putting just enough pull on it to make it straight, then "plucking" it. The rubber band will vibrate at a slow rate. Now if we stretch it tight and pluck it again, the rate of vibration will increase. The mass of the rubber band has remained the same, but as it is stretched tighter, the stiffness has increased (i.e., it becomes proportionally greater). Therefore, for any given system, the greater the stiffness component becomes relative to mass, the higher the rate of vibration.

One vibration is one back-and-forth or one up-and-down excursion. The faster the rate of vibration, the more vibrations occur per unit time, or the more frequently vibrations occur. Thus, the rate of vibration is termed the *frequency of vibration*. Considering these factors, as stiffness becomes proportionally greater than mass, the frequency of vibration increases. Conversely, as mass becomes relatively greater than stiffness, the frequency of vibration decreases. The frequency with which a system vibrates when set into vibration is called its **resonant frequency** (or **natural frequency**).

▼ **Resonant frequency** Frequency at which a system will be most easily set into vibration; point at which the effects of mass and stiffness are equal.

The resonant frequency of a system is determined by the relative magnitude of the mass and stiffness components of its impedance. The resonant frequency is that point at which the effects of mass and stiffness are equal, resulting in total opposition to energy flow determined by resistance alone (Figure 1-16).

Looking at this from a slightly different perspective, any system will respond (i.e., be set into vibration) most readily when stimulated at its resonant frequency. This can be demonstrated in a variety of ways.

If we were to take a set of tuning forks and, one at a time, strike each fork, then place the base of the fork on a table, we would find that the loudness of one fork would increase much more than that of others. The frequency of the tuning fork producing the greatest increase in loudness would be very close to the resonant frequency of the table. This is called **sounding board resonance** (or **sounding board effect**) and occurs because the tabletop is set into vibration, thereby considerably increasing the size of the vibrating surface and creating a source of sound in addition to our tuning fork.

In conducting this experiment, we also note that although the tone becomes louder at the resonant frequency, we hear it for a shorter time than we would if we simply struck the tuning fork and listened to it.

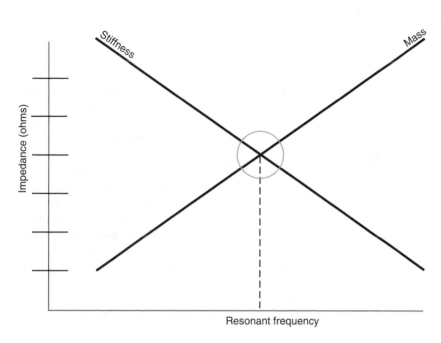

Resonant frequency

Frequency (Hz)

FIG. 1-16

Resonant frequency.

This is caused in part by the increase in resistance afforded by air to vibration of the whole tabletop versus that afforded to the two prongs of the tuning fork. In larger part this is caused by the energy being imparted to the tabletop, resulting in a more rapid use of energy.

The rate at which the magnitude of vibration, and subsequently the loudness of the resultant sound, decreases is called **damping**. When the sound diminishes rapidly, we refer to the system as being *heavily damped;* if it diminishes slowly, it is *lightly damped.*

Using tuning forks with a resonant frequency of vibration that is different from the resonant frequency of the tabletop, we note very little change in loudness as we touch the base of the fork to the tabletop, but the sound will be heard for about as long as if we were not to touch it to the tabletop. This occurs because very little of the original energy is being imparted to the tabletop. That is, the opposition to transfer of energy (the impedance) is large for those frequencies remote from the resonant frequency.

▼ **Damping** Rate at which the magnitude of vibration and the loudness of the resultant sound decreases.

SIDE NOTES

Cavity (Acoustical) Resonance

A standard laboratory demonstration of cavity resonance consists of inserting one end of a straight tube open at both ends into a beaker of water (Figure 1-17).

The end of the tube inserted into the water can be viewed as "closed," and the unsubmerged end is considered "open." A vibrating tuning fork is then placed over the open end of the tube. As the tube is slowly moved up and down in the water, a certain length of tube above the water (its *effective length*) is found that causes an increase in the perceived amplitude of the tuning fork's tone. At this point, the length of tube above the water provides the tube with the same natural frequency of vibration (resonant frequency) as that of the vibrating tuning fork. The vibrations of the tuning fork are exciting the molecules comprising the column of air within the length of tube above the water line. Amplitude becomes maximal (i.e., resonance occurs) when the tube length is such that standing wave patterns representing air molecular velocity (speed) and

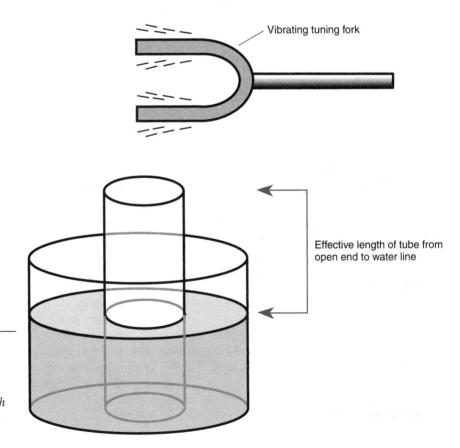

Vibrating tuning fork

Effective length of tube from open end to water line

FIG. 1-17

Laboratory demonstration of resonance. (From Fucci DJ, Lass NJ: *Fundamentals of speech science,* Boston, 1997, Allyn & Bacon.)

pressure (force per unit area) are established within the tube (Figure 1-18, *A* and *B*).

The *standing wave pattern* referring to the velocity (speed) of the air molecules within the tube represents a condition where the molecules are showing *maximum* velocity at the open end of the tube and *minimum* velocity at the closed end of the tube when the tube is being excited by the vibrations of the tuning fork. The speed of movement of the molecules between the extreme ends of the tube follows a curvilinear line (Figure 1-18, *A*). The velocity or speed of air particle movement is in reference to the oscillatory movements of air molecules around a fixed

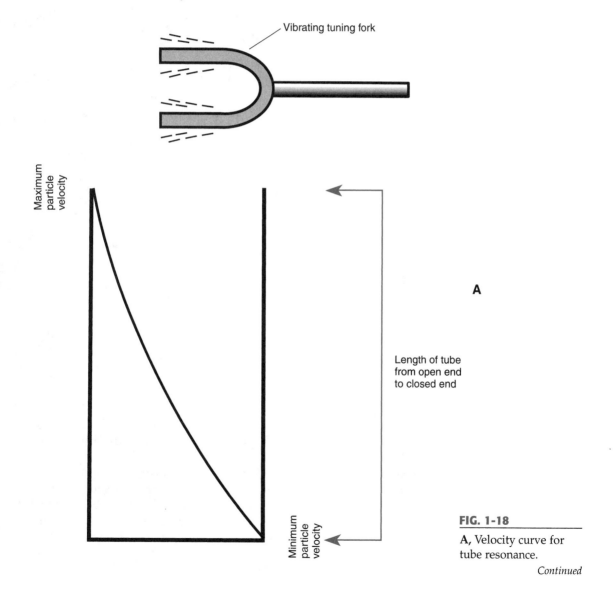

FIG. 1-18

A, Velocity curve for tube resonance.

Continued

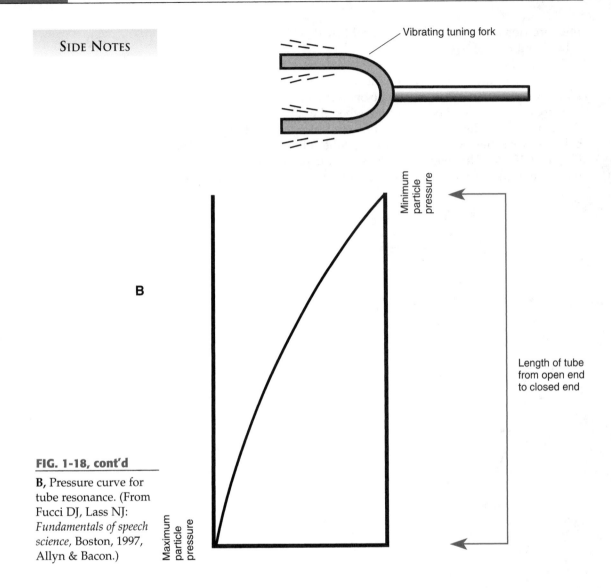

FIG. 1-18, cont'd

B, Pressure curve for tube resonance. (From Fucci DJ, Lass NJ: *Fundamentals of speech science,* Boston, 1997, Allyn & Bacon.)

point. Because of the elastic and inertial properties of the medium, these air particles do not move very far from a fixed point **(rest position)** when they are set in motion.

Sound, which is a disturbance in the particles of a medium, travels through the medium, but the medium's particles remain relatively fixed, allowing the sound disturbance to cause them to oscillate about a fixed point to which they are anchored. Therefore, the speed of the oscillations of the air particles would be *greatest* at the open end of the tube and *least* at the closed end of the tube when the tube is excited by a sound source having the same natural frequency of vibration (resonant frequency) as the tube itself. Tube length, as suggested by the laboratory demonstration in Figure 1-17, appears to be a critical factor in the determination of the natural (resonant) frequencies at which the column of air inside a particular tube will vibrate.

SIDE NOTES

A *pressure* (force per unit area) *curve* can also be drawn to represent molecular activity within the tube when resonance is occurring. The pressure curve shows that while resonance is occurring, there is *minimum* particle pressure at the open end of the tube and *maximum* particle pressure at the closed end of the tube. The pressures on the molecules between the extreme ends follow a curvilinear line (Figure 1-18, *B*).

There appears to be an inverse relationship between the velocity and pressure curves that represent cavity or tube resonance (Figure 1-18). The speed of oscillatory behavior for a particular air molecule is *greatest* at points along the length of the tube where the pressure being applied to that molecule by the vibrating sound source is *least* (i.e., the open end of the tube). Conversely, the speed of oscillatory behavior for a particular air molecule is *least* at points along the length of the tube where the pressure being applied to that molecule by the vibrating sound source is *greatest* (i.e., the closed end of the tube).

If the tuning fork in the laboratory demonstration (see Figure 1-17) had a natural frequency of 500 Hz and was set into vibration over the open end of the tube, careful movement of the tube up and down in the water would show that resonance would occur in the tube when its length from its open end to the water line is 17 cm (Figure 1-19). This length of tube would allow for the establishment of the velocity and pressure standing wave patterns needed for resonance to occur within the tube when the tube is being excited by a 500-Hz sound source (tuning fork).

The speed of molecular movement and the pressure on the air molecules making up the column of air in the tube would be such that the appropriate standing wave patterns would be established. *Tube length,* which has been adjusted to accommodate the excitatory frequency of the tuning fork (500 Hz), is critical to the resonance characteristics of the tube. This is because the tube length needed for resonance to occur is equal to the wavelength (λ) of the frequency of the sound source (the 500-Hz tuning fork) stimulating the tube, divided by a factor of 4, as follows:

$$\text{Tube length} = \frac{\text{Wavelength } (\lambda)}{4}$$

To determine the tube length needed for resonance to occur when it is being excited by a 500-Hz tuning fork, it is first necessary to determine the wavelength of that particular excitatory frequency. Wavelength (λ) is

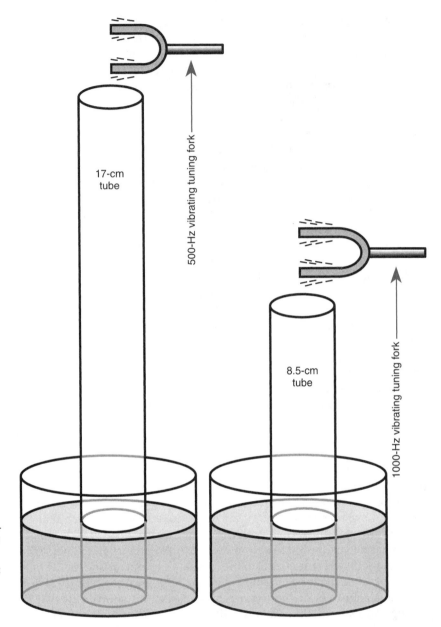

FIG. 1-19

The resonance for tubes of different lengths. (From Fucci DJ, Lass NJ: *Fundamentals of speech science*, Boston, 1997, Allyn & Bacon.)

equal to the speed of sound (velocity) in air (approximately 340 meters per second) divided by the stimulus frequency, as follows:

$$\text{Wavelength } (\lambda) = \frac{\text{Velocity of sound in air}}{\text{Stimulus frequency}}$$

In this specific example, the wavelength for a 500-Hz signal would be 340 meters (or 34,000 cm) per second (velocity of sound in air) divided by 500 Hz (stimulus frequency), which is equal to 0.68 meter (or 68 cm):

$$\text{Wavelength } (\lambda) = \frac{340 \text{ m/sec}}{500 \text{ Hz}} = 0.68 \text{ m} = 68 \text{ cm}$$

Because the tube length needed for resonance to occur is equal to wavelength divided by a factor of 4, a wavelength of 68 cm divided by 4 is equal to a tube length of 17 cm. This is the tube length required for cavity (tube) resonance to occur when the tube is being activated by a tuning fork with a natural (resonant) frequency of vibration of 500 Hz (see Figure 1-19):

$$\text{Tube length} = \frac{68 \text{ cm}}{4} = 17 \text{ cm}$$

If the tuning fork had a natural frequency of vibration of 1000 Hz, the tube length needed for resonance to occur would be 8.5 cm (see Figure 1-19). Wavelength would be equal to 340 meters per second (velocity of sound in air) divided by 1000 Hz (the stimulus frequency), which would be 0.34 m, or 34 cm:

$$\text{Wavelength } (\lambda) = \frac{340 \text{ m/sec}}{1000 \text{ Hz}} = 0.34 \text{ m} = 34 \text{ cm}$$

Thus, the tube length needed for resonance to occur is equal to wavelength divided by a factor of 4, which is 8.5 cm when the tube is being excited by a tuning fork with a natural frequency of 1000 Hz:

$$\text{Tube length} = \frac{34 \text{ cm}}{4} = 8.5 \text{ cm}$$

It would appear from the two previous examples that the shorter (8.5-cm) tube demonstrated a higher resonant frequency (natural frequency of vibration) than the longer (17-cm) tube. As the length of a tube closed at one end and open at the other end (with uniform cross-sectional dimensions throughout its length) is either increased or decreased, its resonance characteristics (i.e., its natural, resonant frequencies) are altered in an orderly pattern. *As tube length is increased, the natural (resonant) frequencies of vibration for the tube become **lower.** Conversely, as tube length is decreased, the natural (resonant) frequencies of vibration for the tube become **higher.***

For example:

$$\text{Tube length} = 15 \text{ cm}$$

$$\text{Wavelength } (\lambda) = 4/1 \times 15 = 60 \text{ cm} \left(\frac{4}{2n - 1} \times L \right)$$

$$f_1 = \text{Velocity/wavelength} = 34{,}000 \text{ cm per sec}/60 \text{ cm} = 567 \text{ Hz}$$

Tube length = 17 cm

Wavelength (λ) = 4/1 × 17 = 68 cm $\left(\dfrac{4}{2n-1} \times L\right)$

f_1 = Velocity/wavelength = 34,000 cm per sec/68 cm = 500 Hz

If tube systems are stimulated by an energy source that contains more than one natural frequency of vibration, multiple resonances will occur simultaneously. In such cases, standing wave patterns are established for each resonant frequency occurring within the tube. The standing wave patterns for the lowest resonant frequency in terms of molecular (particle) velocity and pressure will be the same as those described earlier in the tuning fork examples (see Figure 1-18).

A systematic relationship exists between the resonant frequencies in the tube model being discussed. A straight tube (one that is uniform in cross-sectional dimensions throughout its length) closed at one end and open at the other end can be multiply resonant when excited by a sound source containing more than a single natural frequency of vibration. The first (lowest) resonant frequency for this tube of uniform cross-sectional dimensions throughout its length is equal to the frequency of a sound wave whose wavelength (λ) is four times the length of the tube:

$$f_1 = \frac{velocity}{wavelength}$$

where wavelength = (4 × Tube length).

The tube's other (higher) resonant frequencies are odd-numbered multiples of the lowest resonant frequency. Thus, its second resonant frequency is equal to the frequency of a sound wave whose wavelength is 4/3 times the length of the tube:

$$f_2 = \frac{velocity}{wavelength}$$

where wavelength = (4/3 × Tube length).

The third resonant frequency for this tube is equal to the frequency of a sound wave whose wavelength is 4/5 times the length of the tube:

$$f_3 = \frac{velocity}{wavelength}$$

where wavelength = (4/5 × Tube length).

For example, for a 17-cm tube open at one end and closed at the other end, of uniform cross-sectional dimensions throughout its length (i.e., constant shape):

$$f_1 = \frac{34,000 \text{ cm/sec}}{4/1 \times 17 \text{ cm}} = \frac{34,000 \text{ cm/sec}}{68 \text{ cm}} = 500 \text{ Hz}$$

$$f_2 = \frac{34,000 \text{ cm/sec}}{4/3 \times 17 \text{ cm}} = \frac{34,000 \text{ cm/sec}}{22.7 \text{ cm}} = 1498 \text{ Hz}$$

$$f_3 = \frac{34{,}000 \text{ cm/sec}}{4/5 \times 17 \text{ cm}} = \frac{34{,}000 \text{ cm/sec}}{13.6} = 2500 \text{ Hz}$$

However, once the tube is altered so that it is not uniform in cross-sectional dimensions (i.e., a tube that is not straight), this specific relationship between the resonant frequencies no longer exists.

Thus, resonance is a characteristic of all periodic vibrating systems that enables them to respond strongly to oscillatory disturbances that are the same as their own natural frequencies of vibration. Vibrating systems are capable of ignoring oscillatory disturbances at frequencies that do not match their own natural frequencies of vibration. If a system is excited at its natural (resonant) frequencies (those to which it responds most violently), it is resonating, and the end result is an increase in overall sound pressure level.

Another demonstration of resonance involves blowing across the opening of a bottle. A bottle contains a column of air that has mass and stiffness. Blowing across the neck of the bottle causes the enclosed column of air to vibrate at its resonant frequency. If we now select a tuning fork with a frequency equal (or very close) to that of the air in the bottle, strike it, and hold it close to the bottle's neck, the tone will increase in loudness. This is true because the column of air enclosed in the bottle acts as an additional sound source as it resonates to the sound generated by the tuning fork.

Although this exercise may be less enjoyable than emptying the bottle, it may aid in understanding tubal resonance. In a tube that is closed at one end, the resonant frequency will be one with a wavelength four times the length of the tube. This was discussed in more detail earlier in this chapter.

Frequency Response Curve

Cavities and tubes can serve as resonators because they contain a column of air capable of vibrating at certain frequencies (their resonant or natural frequencies). A graph of the frequencies to which a resonator will respond (resonate) can be constructed; this graph is called a **frequency response curve** (or **resonance curve**).

Undamped resonators are those that resonate to a narrow range of frequencies because they contain only a narrow range of frequencies. Figure 1-20 shows the sharply peaked frequency response curve of an undamped resonator, a tuning fork (which vibrates at only one frequency). *Damped resonators,* on the other hand, resonate to a broad range of frequencies, and as shown in Figure 1-20, they are characterized by a flat, broad frequency response curve. The range of frequencies to which a resonator responds (i.e., the range of a resonator's natural or resonant

▼ **Frequency response curve** Graph of the frequencies to which a resonator will respond.

▼ **Bandwidth** Range of frequencies to which a resonator responds.

frequencies) is called its **bandwidth.** Figure 1-21 shows the derivation of bandwidth. Note that the actual range of frequencies is determined at a point 3 dB below the peak value of the spectrum. This point of measurement is often referred to as the *half power point.*

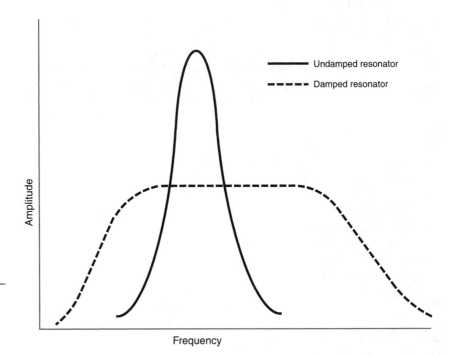

FIG. 1-20

Frequency response curves of undamped and damped resonators.

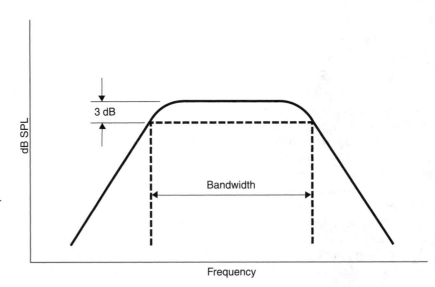

FIG. 1-21

Schematic of how bandwidth is calculated. *dB SPL,* Decibel sound pressure level.

Ear Canal Analogy

The tube model presented earlier is of interest to hearing scientists and audiologists because of its analogy to the human external auditory meatus (Figure 1-22). The human ear canal is bounded laterally by the concha of the auricle and medially by the tympanic membrane. It is analogous to a tube system open at one end (auricle) and closed at its other end (tympanic membrane), and it is relatively uniform (but not straight) in cross-sectional dimensions throughout its length. The ear canal is approximately 2.5 cm in length when measured from the lip of the concha of the auricle to the tympanic membrane. When excited by the sounds being generated by various sound sources, the ear canal responds to those sounds at its own natural (resonant) frequencies. Thus, the human ear canal is similar to a tube closed at one end and open at the other end.

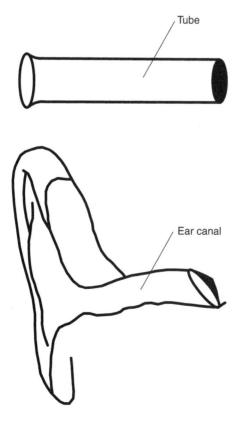

Tube

Ear canal

FIG. 1-22

An inanimate tube compared to the human ear canal.

However, there are differences between an inanimate tube and the human ear canal. Consider the following formula:

$$f_1 = \frac{34,000 \text{ cm/sec}}{4/1 \times 2.5 \text{ cm}} = 3400 \text{ Hz}$$

Research has shown that the average resonant frequency of the external ear canal is approximately 2700 Hz. The discrepancy between this formula and the empirical data probably occurs because the external auditory canal is not straight, does not have uniform dimensions, and is not hard walled. Moreover, the resonant frequency varies considerably from one individual to another. The resonance of the external ear canal provides an increase in sound pressure level for the frequency range of 2000 to 3000 Hz at the tympanic membrane. These frequencies are very important for the perception of the speech signal. Thus, the concept of resonance, particularly cavity (acoustical) resonance, is very important in understanding the human auditory mechanism. These are important considerations for audiologists in many situations, including hearing aid evaluation and interpretation of audiometric data.

THE DECIBEL

In dealing with sound pressure, several problems arise. The first of these pertains to the fact that the only place where there is no sound is in a vacuum. Thus, for practical purposes, there is no "absence of sound." Because there is no "zero" sound pressure, some reference pressure must be determined to represent zero. The reference decided on was the smallest pressure variation from ambient, or atmospheric, pressure produced by a 1-kHz pure tone that could be detected by young listeners with no auditory pathology and who were trained in detection of this acoustic signal. This pressure variation was determined to be 0.0002 dyne/cm². This notation may appear confusing; to review: pressure is measured as force distributed over some given area. The *dyne* is a measure of force, and the square centimeter (cm²) is the size of the area over which the force is distributed. The reference pressure of 0.0002 dyne/cm² is also noted as 0.0002 μbar (microbar), 10 μn/m² (micronerotons per square meter) and, most often today, 20 μPa (written as "twenty micropascals"). This is the basic reference for all sound pressure measurement and is referred to as **physicists' zero.**

As previously described, this reference pressure was determined in reference to human hearing. The ratio of this smallest pressure

▼ **Physicists' zero** Basic reference for all sound pressure measurement; smallest pressure variation from ambient pressure produced by a 1-kHz pure tone that could be detected by young listeners with no auditory pathology and who were trained to detect this signal.

detectable by humans for a 1-kHz tone to the pressure that produces pain is about 10 million to one. The magnitude of this difference precludes direct measurement in terms of dyne/cm², μbar, μn/m², or μPa simply because the number would be too cumbersome (0.0002, 0.0003, etc.) and the measurement increments are much smaller than we need.

To circumvent this problem, a ratio measurement was initiated, which is the ratio of the sound we are interested in measuring to the reference pressure of 0.0002 Pa. This direct ratio measurement also yielded impractically large numbers. For example, conversational speech is normally about 0.5 Pa. The ratio of this pressure to our reference pressure is 2500 (i.e., 0.5 Pa/0.0002 Pa = 2500). Traffic on a noisy street is approximately 2 Pa; the ratio of this noise to our reference is 10,000 (i.e., 2 Pa/ 0.0002 Pa = 10,000). Therefore, it was decided that our measurement of pressure must be based on the logarithm to the base 10 ($\log_{10}$) of this ratio; however, this measurement yielded increments that were much too bulky. That is, $\log_{10}$ of the ratio of conversational speech to our reference pressure is 3.39794, and that of traffic noise is 4.0 (i.e., $\log_{10}$ of 2500 = 3.39794, $\log_{10}$ of 10,000 = 4.0). Subsequently, it was decided that $\frac{1}{10}$ the log of the ratio would be the appropriate measure. To determine $\frac{1}{10}$ the log of the ratio, we multiply the log of the ratio by 10; hence, the equation becomes $10(\log_{10} x/0.0002 \text{ Pa})$. This equation yields a measure of sound power.

For reasons beyond the scope of this chapter, sound pressure is proportional to sound power squared. Again, mathematicians tell us that to square a logarithm, we should double the exponent; that is, $\log_{10}$ of 10 is 1 ($10^1 = 10$), $\log_{10}$ of 100 is 2 ($10^2 = 100$), $\log_{10}$ of 10,000 is 4 ($10^4 = 10,000$), and so on. Therefore, to obtain decibels of sound pressure, we can multiply the $\log_{10}$ of the ratio of the sound we are measuring to our reference pressure of 0.0002 Pa by 20 rather than 10. Our formula for measurement of the pressure parameter of sound is then 20 times the $\log_{10}$ of the ratio of the sound we are measuring to 0.0002 Pa or $20 (\log_{10} \times x/0.0002) = \text{dB}$ SPL. The notation *dB SPL* introduces two abbreviations. The dB is the abbreviation for *decibel,* with the B capitalized in honor of Alexander Graham Bell; SPL stands for *sound pressure level.*

Several important points relate to the way sound is measured. First, the reference pressure was established on the basis of human hearing only at one frequency, 1 kHz. This point becomes important in a later chapter as we discuss how our hearing varies at different frequencies. Another point relates to the decibel as a logarithmic measurement: it requires a much greater increase in sound pressure to increase sound pressure level (SPL) by 1 dB from, for example, 80 to 81 dB SPL than from 20 to 21 dB SPL. The change in sound pressure necessary to increase from 80 to 81 dB SPL is 122 times greater than that necessary to increase 1 dB from 20 to 21 dB SPL.

A Computational Perspective

As previously described, the decibel is a unit of measurement for the amplitude of a signal. It is a ratio scale based on logarithms and is usually used to express ratios between sound pressures. The decibel is an effective means of expressing sound amplitude because of the tremendous range between the weakest sound that humans can hear and the loudest sound that they can tolerate without physical pain. The amplitude ratio of the loudest bearable sound to the faintest audible sound for human hearing is approximately 100,000,000,000,000:1 (100 trillion to one), an extremely large range of numbers. The decibel scale is much more convenient because it provides a much smaller, more manageable range of numbers to use. For example, the ratio of 100,000,000,000,000:1 can be expressed in the decibel scale as a range from *140* (the loudest sound before physical pain) to *1* (the softest sound that can be heard). The key to making this conversion to the smaller range of numbers lies in the use of logarithms. A **logarithm** is a convenient arithmetic shorthand that converts ratio scales into interval scales to reduce the size of the numbers required (Table 1-1).

A *ratio scale* can be represented by the following set of numbers: $\frac{1}{1000}$, $\frac{1}{100}$, $\frac{1}{10}$, 1, 10, 100, 1000, 10,000, 100,000. Each number in the ratio scale can be derived by multiplying the preceding number by 10.

An *interval scale,* representing the same range of numbers as the ratio scale above, can be represented by the following set of numbers: 10^{-3}, 10^{-2}, 10^{-1}, 10^{0}, 10^{1}, 10^{2}, 10^{3}, 10^{4}, 10^{5}. The superscript number *(exponent)* in the scale tells us how many times 10 must be multiplied by itself to obtain the equivalent number in the ratio scale. For example, 10^{2} (10 to the second power) indicates that $10 \times 1 = 10$, $\times 10 = 100$, which is the ratio scale equivalent of 10^{2}; 10 to the third power (10^{3}) shows that $10 \times 1 = 10$, $\times 10 = 100$, $\times 10 = 1000$, which is the ratio scale equivalent of 10^{3}. The number 10, therefore, is assumed to be a base that can be raised to some power to represent larger numbers on a ratio scale. The *exponents* to

TABLE 1-1.	Logarithms (Exponents) to Base 10	
Desired Number	**Base 10**	**Logarithm**
10	10	1
100	10×10	2
1000	$10 \times 10 \times 10$	3
10,000	$10 \times 10 \times 10 \times 10$	4
100,000	$10 \times 10 \times 10 \times 10 \times 10$	5
1,000,000	$10 \times 10 \times 10 \times 10 \times 10 \times 10$	6

which the base is raised are logarithms. The range of numbers from $\frac{1}{1000}$ to 100,000 can be represented by the smaller set of logarithms ranging from –3 to 5, with the assumption being that the base for the interval scale is 10.

The *Bel* is an arbitrary logarithmic unit used to represent sound amplitude on an interval scale. Bel is a mathematical term defining the logarithm of a ratio; in the 1960s it was capitalized in honor of Alexander Graham Bell (1847–1922). (Although Bell is most famous for the invention of the telephone, he was also a deaf educator and created one of the earliest symbol systems for teaching deaf persons to communicate.)

$$Bel = \log_{10} x/\text{reference}$$

As previously stated, the ratio between the weakest sound we can detect and the loudest sound we can tolerate before feeling physical pain is 100,000,000,000,000:1 (100 trillion to one). This range of sound amplitude can be represented by a factor of "14 Bels." The logarithm (to the base 10) of 100,000,000,000,000 is 14; 10 raised to the fourteenth power (10^{14}) is equal to 100,000,000,000,000 (100 trillion). The problem with the Bel is that it provides too few units (14) to represent the tremendous sound amplitude range available to human ears. Consequently, the decibel (dB) is used; it is one tenth of a Bel. If 1 Bel is equal to 10 dB, the range of human hearing can be represented by 140 dB, which seems to be a convenient interval scale size for expressing sound amplitudes.

The logarithm of a number can be determined through the use of log tables, which can be found in most statistics books, or through the use of a scientific calculator, which usually has a "log" key. It is assumed that the log key on the calculator represents a log scale to the base 10, unless specified otherwise. In the previous examples, the logarithm of the numbers involved could be determined by counting zeroes: the log of 1000 is 3; the log of 10 is 1; and so forth.

Sound amplitudes are usually determined by the amount of pressure (force per unit area) that they are causing to occur on a thin plate or diaphragm. On the inside of a microphone or the receiver end of a telephone, there is a thin disk that moves in accordance with the sound pressure impinging on it. The scale most often used to measure sound amplitude is the **sound pressure level (SPL)** scale. This scale measures amplitudes in terms of dynes/cm^2 or pascals (Pa). The reference point for this scale is 0.0002 dyne/cm^2 (20 µPa), which, as mentioned earlier, is roughly equivalent to the weakest sound amplitude that humans can detect at 1000 Hz. The formula for expressing dB ratios when using the SPL scale involves multiplying the logarithm of the sound amplitude ratios by 20 (instead of 10, as used for expressing dB ratios in intensity levels). The reason for this change is because intensity is proportional to

▼ **Sound pressure level**
Scale used to measure sound amplitude in terms of dynes/cm^2 or pascals (Pa).

pressure squared ($I = P^2$). The formula for expressing dB ratios when using the sound pressure level scale is as follows:

$$dB\ SPL = 20 \log (P_1/P_2)$$

where *SPL* = sound pressure level; *20* = a constant; P_1 = higher sound pressure; and P_2 = lower sound pressure. The box provides examples of how this formula works.

> *SPL Example 1: If one sound amplitude is 1000 times greater than another sound amplitude, the dB difference on the sound pressure level scale is 60 dB SPL (dB SPL = 20 × log 1000/1; 1000 divided by 1 = 1000; the logarithm of 1000 [to the base 10] = 3; 20 × 3 = 60 dB SPL).*

> *SPL Example 2: If one sound amplitude is 50 dynes/cm² (Pa) and another sound amplitude is 5 dynes/cm² (Pa), the dB difference on the sound pressure level scale is 20 dB SPL (dB SPL = 20 × log 50 dynes per cm² (Pa)/5 dynes per cm² (Pa); 50 divided by 5 = 10; the logarithm of 10 [to the base 10] = 1; 20 × 1 = 20 dB SPL).*

▼ **Hearing level** Scale used by audiologists in which the zero point represents normal human hearing and is different for each frequency.

When testing hearing, audiologists use a measurement scale that is an offshoot of the sound pressure level scale. They use the **hearing level (HL)** or **hearing threshold level (HTL)** scale. The zero point for this scale is elevated from the bottom of the SPL scale (0.0002 dynes/cm² [Pa]). The HL scale represents normal human hearing and is different for each frequency tested because human hearing does not show the same sensitivity for each frequency. For example, at 1000 Hz, 0 dB HL is set at approximately 7.5 dB SPL. At this frequency, the average normal listener would just begin to hear a pure tone at 7.5 dB SPL.

Audiologists have developed the HL scale to use a scale in which the "0" represents median hearing sensitivity for normal-hearing young adults. For example, a child who has had little exposure to loud sounds or extreme environmental noises, plus a small ear canal volume, could have a hearing level value of –5 dB HL at 1000 Hz. The HL scale has been adjusted from time to time as hearing scientists and audiologists have adopted different zero values based on more recent research findings.

SUMMARY

The physics of sound includes the conditions necessary to create sound, properties of vibrating systems, simple harmonic motion, sine curves and their spatial and temporal features, Fourier analysis, the spectral analysis of complex periodic and aperiodic sounds, resonance and its importance in hearing, and the decibel. An understanding of these concepts will assist the reader in applying basic concepts in acoustics to an understanding of audition.

The pure tone is the basic component of all sound. The pure tone, represented graphically by a sine curve, provides a representation of the two basic parameters of sound: time and pressure. We rarely encounter pure tones in our daily lives; rather, we hear complex sounds with overall quality affected by component pure tones and their temporal (phase) relationships as well as the acoustic environment, including reflection, absorption, and resonance. Time and pressure parameters can be quantified as frequency (Hz) and sound pressure level (dB), respectively, and these physical parameters can be related to human hearing.

It is important to keep these points in mind as we discuss the auditory system and psychoacoustics. The complex perception of acoustic events that serves us so well depends on the physical parameters of sound, the physiology of the auditory system, and psychological factors of sound association. Some understanding of each of these areas is necessary to form a concept of how we couple the physical stimulus to our reactions.

SUGGESTED READINGS

Durant JD, Lovrinic JH: *Bases of hearing science*, ed 3, Philadelphia, 1995, Lippincott Williams & Wilkins.

Fucci DJ, Lass NJ: *Fundamentals of speech science*, Boston, 1997, Allyn & Bacon.

Raphael LJ, Borden GJ, Harris KS: *Speech science primer: physiology, acoustics, and perception of speech*, ed 5, Philadelphia, 2006, Lippincott Williams & Wilkins.

Speaks CE: *Introduction to sound: acoustics for the hearing and speech sciences*, ed 3, San Diego, 2000, Singular.

Yost WA: *Fundamentals of hearing: an introduction*, ed 5, San Diego, 2006, Academic Press.

STUDY QUESTIONS

True-False

_____1. Hertz (Hz) is a unit of measurement for wavelength.

_____2. White noise has energy distributed evenly over a wide band of frequencies.

_____3. The decibel scale is a linear scale.

_____4. A medium that returns to its original shape is said to possess elasticity.

_____5. Resistance causes a vibrating body to remain in motion.

_____6. For resonance to occur in a tube, the tube length must be half the wavelength of the resonant frequency.

Fill in the Blank

1. A sound that has almost all its energy located at a single frequency is a _____.

2. A wave shape that does not repeat itself as a function of time is a _____ sound disturbance.

3. The process of changing energy from one form to another is _____.

4. When testing hearing, audiologists use the _____ scale.

5. A graph showing amplitude as a function of frequency is called a _____.

Matching

Match the following terms (a-g) with the definitions (1-7).
a. Amplitude
b. Impedance
c. Reverberation
d. Decibel
e. Sound
f. Pitch
g. Inertia

_____1. A condition of disturbance of particles in a medium.

_____2. A body in motion remains in motion.

_____3. Maximum displacement of particles in a medium.

_____4. The perceptual correlate of frequency.

_____5. Unit of measurement of amplitude of a signal.

_____6. Repeated reflection of sound.

_____7. Opposition to flow of energy.

STRUCTURE AND FUNCTION

ANATOMY AND PHYSIOLOGY OF THE CONDUCTIVE AUDITORY MECHANISM

KEY TERMS

Peripheral auditory system
Central auditory system
Outer ear
Middle ear

Inner ear
Conductive mechanism
Sensory mechanism
Central mechanism
Temporal bone
Air cells
Auricle (pinna)
External auditory meatus (outer ear canal)
Tympanic membrane (eardrum)
Cerumen
Annulus
Tympanic sulcus
Pars tensa
Pars flaccida (Shrapnell's membrane)
Umbo
Cone of light
Malleus
Quadrants
Fenestra vestibuli
Fenestra rotunda
Promontory
Cranial nerve VII (facial nerve)
Chorda tympani
Pyramidal eminence
Stapedius muscle
Tensor tympani muscle
Temporal bone
Tympanic cavity proper (tympanum)
Epitympanic recess (attic)
Auditory (eustachian) tube
Ossicles (ossicular chain)
Incus
Stapes
Cranial nerve V (trigeminal nerve)
Labyrinthine wall
Perilymph
Impedance
Middle ear transformer
Condensation effect (areal ratio)
Curved-membrane buckling mechanism
Ostium
Conductive hearing loss
Acoustic reflex

LEARNING OBJECTIVES:

After studying this chapter, the student will be able to do the following:

1. Identify and describe the two subsystems of the human auditory system.
2. Discuss the three main functional mechanisms of the peripheral auditory system.
3. Define the major structures that compose the outer ear and discuss how each structure functions in the auditory system.
4. Identify the three layers of tissue and two types of fibers that make up the tympanic membrane.
5. Describe the structure of the middle ear.
6. Identify the specific nerves and muscles that appear in the middle ear.
7. Describe the differences between the epitympanic recess (attic) and the tympanic cavity proper (tympanum).
8. Describe the ossicular chain and identify the three ossicles in the middle ear.
9. Discuss the functions of the auricle and external auditory meatus in the conductive auditory mechanism.
10. Describe the auditory mechanism in terms of energy conduction.
11. Define impedance.
12. Discuss the effects of atmospheric pressure on the auditory system and potential complications of differential pressure.
13. Describe the three functions of the auditory tube.
14. Discuss the effects of the muscles surrounding the middle ear in terms of acoustic reflex.

The human auditory system can be divided anatomically into two subsystems: the **peripheral auditory system** and the **central auditory system**. It can be further subdivided anatomically into four divisions: the **outer ear,** the **middle ear,** the **inner ear,** and the **central auditory system.** Functionally, the auditory system is composed of three main components: the **conductive mechanism,** the **sensory mechanism,** and the **central mechanism** (Figure 2-1).

Almost all of the peripheral auditory mechanism is located in the **temporal bone,** a paired cranial bone of the skull that comprises the major portion of the lateral base and sides of the *braincase* (Figure 2-2, *A*). Each temporal bone consists of four portions (Figure 2-2, *B* and *C*). The *squamous portion* contains the opening of the *external auditory meatus* (outer ear canal). The *mastoid portion* is behind the auricle and contains

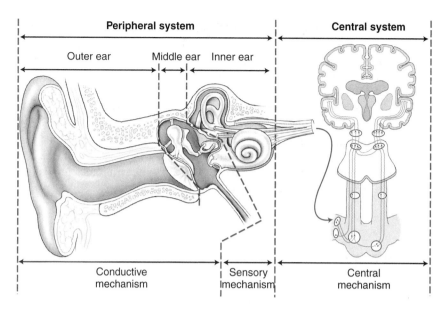

SIDE NOTES

FIG. 2-1

Anatomical and functional divisions of the auditory mechanism.

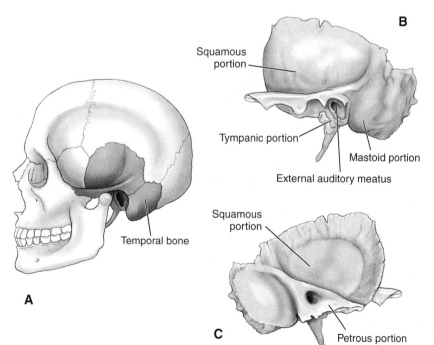

FIG. 2-2

A, Temporal bone in the skull. **B,** Left temporal bone, lateral view. **C,** Left temporal bone, medial view.

SIDE NOTES

numerous air-filled spaces **(air cells).** Part of the *tympanic portion* forms a section of the *external auditory meatus.* The *petrous portion* is located at the base of the skull and houses the essential parts of the organs of hearing and equilibrium.

The anatomy of the conductive auditory mechanism includes the outer ear and middle ear (see Figure 2-1). Its function is to *conduct* sound energy from the outside environment to the inner ear. This process includes a natural amplification and impedance matching that contribute dramatically to normal auditory sensitivity. It also contains two muscles that may filter sound, particularly at higher intensity levels and during times of stress to the organism.

OUTER EAR

▼ **Outer ear** Outermost portion of the auditory system, consisting of the auricle and external auditory meatus.

The outer ear represents the outermost portion of the auditory system and consists of the **auricle** (or **pinna**) and the **external auditory meatus** (or **outer ear canal**).

Auricle (Pinna)

▼ **Auricle** Outermost portion of the auditory system, forming a cup around the entrance to the external auditory meatus.

The auricle is the outermost portion of the conductive (and overall auditory) mechanism (Figure 2-3). It is composed of soft tissue and cartilage that form a "cup" around the entrance to the external auditory meatus, and its skin is continuous with the skin of the meatus.

The surface of the auricle is uneven and contains pits, depressions, ridges, and grooves. The *concha* is the deepest depression on the auricle; it leads directly to and forms the opening of the external auditory meatus. The *helix* is the rimlike ridge on the periphery of the auricle that begins just superior to the opening of the external auditory meatus and runs around much of the periphery of the auricle. The ridge just inside the helix, called the *antihelix,* follows a similar course as the helix. Depressions on the auricle include the *scaphoid fossa* (which lies between the helix and antihelix) and the *triangular fossa* (which is medial to the scaphoid fossa in the superior portion of the auricle between the helix and antihelix). The *tragus* is a small flap of cartilage on the anterior wall of the external auditory meatus. The *antitragus* lies just opposite the tragus and forms the inferior boundary of the concha. The most inferior landmark on the auricle is the *lobule (lobe);* it is composed of soft tissue and is highly vascular.

Although in some species, including cats and dogs, the auricle may help to collect and direct sound energy into the external auditory

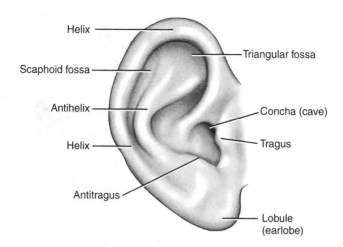

Helix

Triangular fossa

Scaphoid fossa

Antihelix

Concha (cave)

Helix

Tragus

Antitragus

Lobule
(earlobe)

SIDE NOTES

FIG. 2-3

Landmarks of the
auricle.

meatus, its function is limited in humans because it cannot be moved toward a sound source independently of the head. Its musculature is vestigial and of limited functional usefulness.

External Auditory Meatus (Outer Ear Canal)

The **external auditory meatus** (outer ear canal) is a canal in the temporal bone lined with a thin skin layer that begins at the concha of the auricle. It is 25 to 35 mm in length, very narrow (5-9 mm in diameter), and serves as a channel that leads to the **tympanic membrane (eardrum),** which is located at the canal's medial end. Figure 2-4 depicts structures in addition to the conductive mechanism in order to provide perspective relative to structures discussed later. The external auditory meatus protects the tympanic membrane from the outside atmosphere. Usually the canal is not perfectly straight but is somewhat S shaped, increasing this protective aspect. As a result, the tympanic membrane usually cannot be seen by looking into the canal unless the auricle is pulled superiorly and posteriorly so that the canal is straightened for viewing the membrane. The lateral one third of the canal, the portion toward the auricle, is composed of cartilage, whereas the medial two thirds (toward the tympanic membrane) contains bone.

Two sets of *glands, ceruminous* (wax secreting) and *sebaceous* (oil producing), line the skin of the cartilaginous portion of the canal. The glandular tissue located within the walls of the external auditory meatus produces a wax called **cerumen.** Along with the oil produced by the sebaceous glands, cerumen keeps the canal supple and clean and reduces dryness. The cartilaginous portion of the canal nearest the

▼ **External auditory meatus** Canal leading from the auricle to the tympanic membrane, approximately 25 to 35 mm long, rather narrow, and S shaped.

▼ **Cerumen** Wax produced by the ceruminous glands in the external auditory meatus that helps to keep the canal clean.

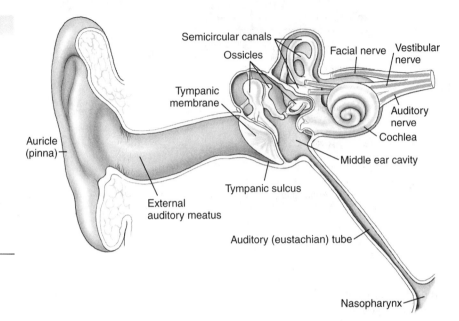

FIG. 2-4

Basic anatomy of the ear: structures of the outer, middle, and inner ear.

auricle is also lined with hairs. Along with cerumen, hairs provide protection for the tympanic membrane against insects and other foreign bodies.

The outer ear mechanism (auricle and external auditory meatus) receives and directs airborne sound to reach the tympanic membrane. Once the acoustic signal reaches this membrane, the sound is converted into mechanical vibrations of the membrane itself.

Tympanic Membrane (Eardrum)

▼ **Tympanic membrane**
Elastic structure that separates the outer ear from the middle ear cavity.

The tympanic membrane is a thin and very elastic membranous structure that separates the external auditory meatus of the outer ear from the middle ear cavity (Figure 2-5). It is surrounded by fibrous tissue called the **annulus,** which fits tightly into the **tympanic sulcus,** a groove in the bony wall of the external auditory meatus (see Figure 2-4). The tympanic membrane varies in individuals from almost transparent to barely translucent (letting light pass through). The tympanic membrane is normally concave and composed of three layers of tissue: (1) an outer, *cutaneous layer* that is continuous with the lining of the external auditory meatus; (2) a middle, *fibrous layer* that is primarily responsible for the compliance of the membrane; and (3) an inner, *mucous membrane layer* that is continuous with the lining of the middle ear cavity. The tympanic membrane also contains two types of fibers: (1) *radial fibers,* which originate near the center of the tympanic membrane (where they are dense)

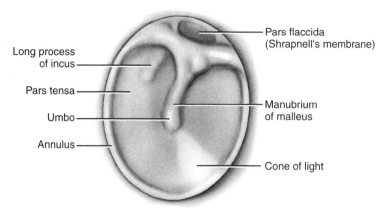

Long process of incus —

Pars tensa —

Umbo —

Annulus —

Pars flaccida (Shrapnell's membrane)

Manubrium of malleus

Cone of light

FIG. 2-5

Tympanic membrane (eardrum).

and spread toward the periphery (where they are sparse), and (2) *circular fibers*, which surround the membrane and are sparse near the center and dense toward the periphery.

The **pars tensa** is the largest portion of the tympanic membrane, containing numerous fibers that contribute to the taut nature of this part of the membrane. In contrast, the **pars flaccida** (also called **Shrapnell's membrane**) is a small triangular area on the superior portion of the membrane that contains very few fibers and therefore is flaccid. The **umbo** is the center point of the tympanic membrane, representing the projection from the *manubrium* of the malleus. The **cone of light** (a reflected spot of light) radiates from the umbo toward the periphery of the tympanic membrane when it is viewed with an *otoscope* (Figure 2-6) or videotoscope, a closed-circuit television that provides visual motion and still photographs of the external ear canal and tympanic membrane.

The **malleus,** the most lateral bone of the ossicular chain in the middle ear, is attached to the fibrous layer of the tympanic membrane and

SIDE NOTES

▼ **Pars tensa** Largest portion of the tympanic membrane, consisting of fibers that contribute to the taut nature of the membrane.

▼ **Pars flaccida** Small section on the superior portion of the tympanic membrane that contains few fibers and is flaccid.

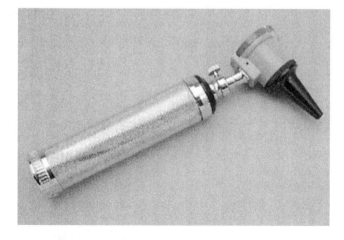

FIG. 2-6

An otoscope. (From Zakus SM: *Mosby's clinical skills for medical assistants,* ed 4, 2001, Mosby.

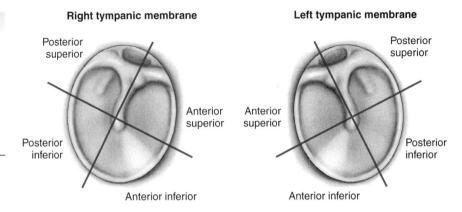

Right tympanic membrane

Posterior superior

Anterior superior

Posterior inferior

Anterior inferior

Left tympanic membrane

Posterior superior

Anterior superior

Posterior inferior

Anterior inferior

FIG. 2-7

Division of the tympanic membrane into quadrants.

is responsible for pulling the tympanic membrane medially toward the middle ear, thus causing its concave shape when viewed from the external auditory meatus. The tympanic membrane is divided into four **quadrants:** *anterior superior, anterior inferior, posterior superior,* and *posterior inferior* (Figure 2-7).

MIDDLE EAR

Airborne sound is transduced to mechanical energy as a result of the collection of sound energy by the tympanic membrane and subsequent movement of the three tiny ossicles within the middle ear. The adult middle ear is a hollow, air-filled cavity approximately 0.5 inch high and wide and about 0.25 inch in depth (lateral to medial) located medial to (behind) the tympanic membrane.

The most medial portion of the middle ear cavity separates the middle ear from the inner ear (Figure 2-8). It contains two openings into the inner ear: the **fenestra vestibuli** (oval window) and the smaller **fenestra rotunda** (round window), which lies inferior to it. It also contains the **promontory,** a bump below the fenestra rotunda that allows extra room on the inner ear side for the first turn of the inner ear's cochlea. Superior to the fenestra vestibuli is **cranial nerve VII (facial nerve)** as it passes through the middle ear. The **chorda tympani,** a branch of the facial nerve, passes through the middle ear (between the ossicles) and carries information about the sense of taste from the anterior portion of the tongue to the central nervous system. The lateral side of the middle ear cavity is formed largely by the tympanic membrane, as well as a section of bone superior to the membrane in the epitympanic recess (attic) region of the middle ear cavity.

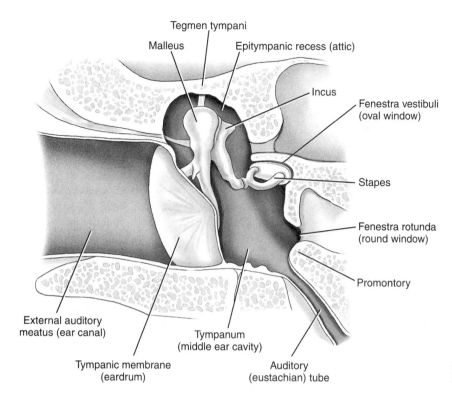

Tegmen tympani
Malleus
Epitympanic recess (attic)
Incus
Fenestra vestibuli (oval window)
Stapes
Fenestra rotunda (round window)
Promontory
External auditory meatus (ear canal)
Tympanum (middle ear cavity)
Tympanic membrane (eardrum)
Auditory (eustachian) tube

FIG. 2-8

Middle ear.

The posterior side of the middle ear cavity contains the **pyramidal eminence,** in which lies the middle ear's **stapedius muscle,** one of two middle ear muscles (Figure 2-9). The **tensor tympani muscle** is contained within a small cavity in that portion of the **temporal bone** that forms the anterior side of the middle ear cavity (Figure 2-10).

The middle ear cavity is divided into two areas: the **tympanic cavity proper** (or **tympanum**) and the **epitympanic recess** (or **attic**) (Figure 2-11). In the inferior, medial portion of the tympanic cavity lies the orifice (internal opening) to the **auditory (eustachian) tube,** which is approximately 35 mm long in the adult and connects the middle ear cavity to the *nasopharynx,* the superior portion of the *pharynx (throat)* just above the *velum (soft palate).* Although the auditory tube is usually in a closed position, the muscles of the nasopharynx open it during swallowing, yawning, and sneezing.

Tympanic Cavity Proper (Tympanum)

The tympanic cavity proper is in the direct line of vision of the tympanic membrane and lies between the membrane and the inner ear (see Figure 2-11). It is filled with air from the auditory (eustachian) tube. Three small

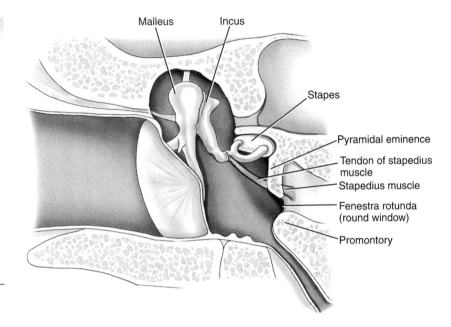

Malleus   Incus

Stapes

Pyramidal eminence

Tendon of stapedius
muscle

Stapedius muscle

Fenestra rotunda
(round window)

Promontory

FIG. 2-9

Location of the
stapedius muscle.

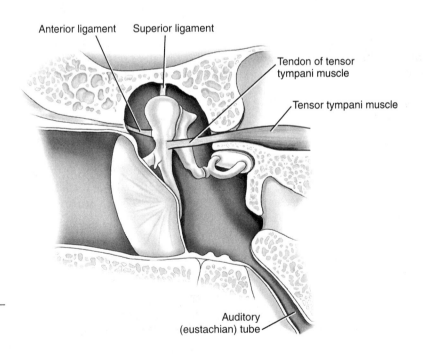

Anterior ligament   Superior ligament

Tendon of tensor
tympani muscle

Tensor tympani muscle

Auditory
(eustachian) tube

FIG. 2-10

Location of the tensor
tympani muscle.

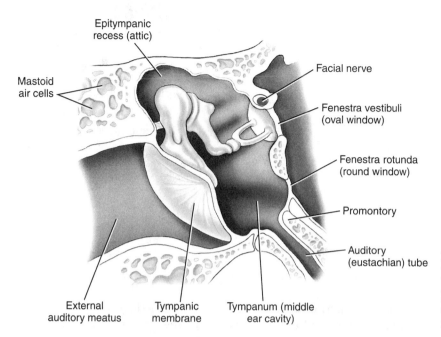

Epitympanic
recess (attic)

Facial nerve

Mastoid
air cells

Fenestra vestibuli
(oval window)

Fenestra rotunda
(round window)

Promontory

Auditory
(eustachian) tube

External
auditory meatus

Tympanic
membrane

Tympanum (middle
ear cavity)

FIG. 2-11

Middle ear divisions of
the tympanic cavity
proper (tympanum)
and the epitympanic
recess (attic).

bones (the smallest in the human body) called the ossicles (or **ossicular chain**) cross the middle ear cavity from its lateral wall to its medial wall for the purpose of transmitting the vibrations of the tympanic membrane to the inner ear mechanism, where the sensory end organ of hearing is located. The first ossicle, the *malleus* (described earlier), is attached to the tympanic membrane; the second is the **incus,** which is attached to the malleus. The **stapes,** the third bone, is attached to the incus, and its footplate inserts into the fenestra vestibuli (oval window), which connects the ossicular chain to the inner ear mechanism (cochlea). The ossicles are held in place by ligaments (see Figure 2-10).

Normally the ossicles vibrate in synchrony with the tympanic membrane and transmit vibrations of the membrane faithfully into the inner ear mechanism. Their Latin names indicate the structures that they resemble: *malleus* = hammer; *incus* = anvil (which is used by blacksmiths); *stapes* = stirrup (like the stirrup on a saddle). Joining the ossicles to each other are joints: the malleus and incus articulate with each other through the *incudomalleolar joint,* and the incus and stapes articulate through the *incudostapedial joint* (Figure 2-12).

Malleus

The malleus, the most lateral of the three ossicles, is attached to the tympanic membrane. It consists of a head, neck, and three processes: the

▼ **Ossicles** Three small bones (malleus, incus, stapes) that cross the middle ear cavity and transmit vibrations from the tympanic membrane to the inner ear.

SIDE NOTES

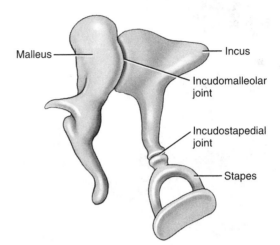

FIG. 2-12

Ossicular chain and connecting joints.

manubrium, anterior process, and lateral process (Figure 2-13). The *head* occupies the space of approximately half the epitympanic recess. The *manubrium* is the portion of the malleus that connects directly to the tympanic membrane and is visible on otoscopic examination of the ear (see Figure 2-5). The *neck* is a constriction between the manubrium and the head. Located at the juncture of the manubrium and the neck is the spinelike *anterior process*. The *lateral process* lies below the anterior process and, as its name indicates, is directed laterally. Because the manubrium of the malleus is attached directly to the tympanic membrane, and because the ossicles are attached to each other, when the tympanic membrane vibrates, the ossicles vibrate in synchrony with the tympanic membrane.

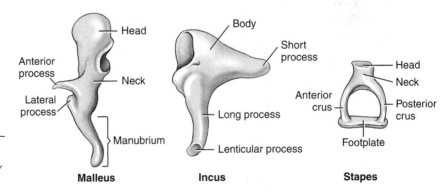

FIG. 2-13

Anatomy of the ossicles: malleus, incus, and stapes.

Incus

The incus consists of a body (which is attached to the head of the malleus) and two processes: a short process and a long process (see Figure 2-13). The *body* and *short process* occupy space in the epitympanic recess, and the *long process* courses vertically downward and is almost parallel to the manubrium of the malleus (see Figure 2-11). Inferiorly, the end of the long process terminates as a rounded projection called the *lenticular process*, which is the portion of the incus that articulates directly with the head of the stapes by means of the incudostapedial joint (see Figure 2-12).

Stapes

The stapes consists of a head, neck, crura, and footplate (see Figure 2-13). The *head* is the most superior portion of the stapes and contains an articular facet for reception of the lenticular process of the incus. The *neck* is a constriction between the head and the two *crura* (*anterior crus* and *posterior crus*). The *crura* connect the neck to the *footplate*, which lies in the fenestra vestibuli (oval window) of the *labyrinthine wall* (medial wall of middle ear cavity) and is held in place by means of an *annular ligament*. Because the fenestra vestibuli couples the middle ear to the inner ear, when the ossicular chain moves, the footplate movement inside the fenestra vestibuli causes movement of the fluid in the inner ear.

Middle Ear Muscles

There are two small muscles in the middle ear, the tensor tympani and stapedius. These are the smallest striated muscles in the human body, which is appropriate because they attach to the smallest bones in the body. The *stapedius* is located in the posterior portion of the middle ear cavity and connects to the neck of the stapes by means of a tendon (see Figure 2-9). On contraction, the neck of the stapes is displaced in the posterior direction. This muscle is innervated by a branch of cranial nerve VII (facial nerve). When the stapedius muscle contracts in response to external sounds, this phenomenon is called the *acoustic reflex*. The *tensor tympani* muscle is located in the anterior portion of the middle ear cavity. It is connected to the manubrium of the malleus (near its neck) by means of a tendon (see Figure 2-10). On contraction, it moves the malleus medially and anteriorly and thus tenses the tympanic membrane. The tensor tympani is innervated by a branch of **cranial nerve V (trigeminal nerve)** and possibly other cranial nerves.

FUNCTION OF THE CONDUCTIVE MECHANISM

Nonacoustic Function

The auricle (pinna) is the outermost portion of the conductive mechanism and, in humans, provides limited acoustic advantage. As mentioned earlier, in some species the auricle helps to collect and direct sound into the external auditory meatus; however, its function is limited in that capacity in humans. Usually the human auricle cannot be directed toward a sound source independently of the head.

The external auditory meatus serves to protect the tympanic membrane from the outside atmosphere in several ways. Usually the canal is not perfectly straight but is somewhat S shaped, providing some protection to the membrane. In addition, the skin of the cartilaginous portion of the canal has two sets of glands: ceruminous and sebaceous. The ceruminous gland produces a wax (lubricant) called **cerumen,** which keeps the canal supple and clean and reduces dryness. Cerumen may also serve as an insect repellent. To prevent cerumen from accumulating to the point of obstructing the external auditory meatus, tiny hairs move the cerumen laterally with a ciliary action. The lateral cartilaginous portion of the canal is also lined with hairs, which provide additional protection for the tympanic membrane against insects and other foreign bodies.

Acoustic Function

The primary function of the conductive mechanism is to *conduct* sound energy from outside the head, through the outer ear and middle ear, to be used by the sensorineural mechanisms. The outer ear mechanism (auricle and external auditory meatus) receives airborne sound and serves as a channel for that sound to reach the tympanic membrane. As described in Chapter 1, the external auditory meatus also provides natural amplification for some sounds by acting as a closed-tube resonator. Its resonant frequency averages approximately 2700 Hz, with considerable variability among individuals. This is clearly a significant advantage in that these frequencies are among the most important for the perception of speech.

Although the average resonance of the external auditory canal amounts to 10 to 15 dB at approximately 2700 Hz, both the resonant frequency and the amount of gain are variable. Some people show as much as 30 dB of gain, and the resonant frequency may be 2000 Hz to 3500 Hz and beyond. Clinically, canal resonance has important implications. First, when hearing is tested under earphones, canal resonance is reduced or eliminated, making thresholds obtained in this manner somewhat questionable as a predictor of auditory sensitivity in our normal condition of movement without earphones. Second, when an ear mold is placed in an ear for fitting a hearing aid, canal resonance is reduced or eliminated, a phenomenon referred to as *insertion loss*. This phenomenon must be taken into consideration in determining how much gain a person needs in a hearing aid.

Once the airborne acoustic signal reaches the tympanic membrane, it is converted into mechanical vibrations of the membrane itself by setting the membrane into vibration. Moreover, the signal remains in a mechanical mode as it is transmitted through the middle ear mechanism. The conductive mechanism is a functional division of the peripheral auditory system that allows sound wave energy to be *conducted* to and through the outer ear and middle ear.

When sound wave energy passes the auricle and moves through the external auditory meatus, it strikes the tympanic membrane, causing the membrane to vibrate. Thus, the acoustic energy of the sound wave is transduced (converted) to mechanical energy through the ossicular chain because the malleus, the first of the three ossicles, is attached (at its manubrium) to the tympanic membrane, the incus is attached to the malleus, and the stapes is attached to the incus (see Figure 2-11). The malleus and incus act as a unit and vibrate in conjunction with the motion of the tympanic membrane. The incus, in turn, passes the energy along to the stapes, whose footplate is attached to the fenestra vestibuli (oval window) on the **labyrinthine wall**, the medial wall that separates the middle ear and inner ear. The stapes' footplate moves in and out of the fenestra vestibuli as it is rocked by the movement of the incus (to which it is attached at its head), thereby transferring the mechanical energy from the middle ear to the inner ear through the fenestra vestibuli.

SIDE NOTES

▼ **Labyrinthine wall** Medial wall of the middle ear that separates it from the inner ear.

Impedance

The footplate of the stapes rests in the fenestra vestibuli, contacting the very dense fluid of the inner ear called **perilymph**. As with all fluids, perilymph has very high **impedance** (opposition to energy flow by a medium). When sound reaches a high-impedance medium, little is absorbed, with the majority reflected away. Conversely, when a sound wave reaches a low-impedance medium, such as air, most of its energy is absorbed by (passes into) that medium. Therefore, when sound needs to flow from a low-impedance medium (air) to a high-impedance medium (water), much of its energy will be reflected away, and only a small amount will be transferred. This impedance mismatch is obvious to anyone who has tried to communicate with another person while that person is underwater. Figure 2-14 provides an example of impedance.

Recall from Chapter 1 that the impedance of any medium is determined by three characteristics of the medium: *mass*, *stiffness*, and *resistance*. An increase in any one of these three characteristics causes a reduction

▼ **Impedance** Opposition to energy flow by a medium.

SIDE NOTES

FIG. 2-14

Example of impedance
mismatch between air
and water. (From
Deutsch LJ, Richards
AM: *Elementary hearing
science,* Boston, 1979,
Allyn & Bacon.)

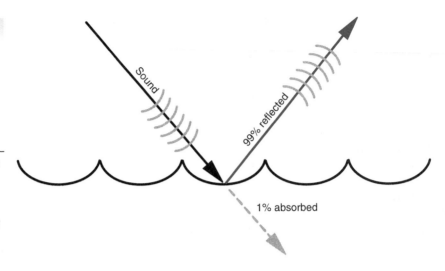

in the flow of sound into a medium (reduced absorption), which
increases the amount of reflected sound.

Impedance Mismatch

The impedance of a normal, air-filled middle ear system is very low.
Each of the factors that contributes to the impedance of the middle
ear (mass of ossicles and tympanic membrane; stiffness and friction of
ossicular joints; stiffness of ossicular chain) are extremely small.

However, when sound energy transported by the low-impedance
middle ear system encounters the high-impedance inner ear fluids,
much energy would be lost if not for the impedance-matching function
of the middle ear. The *impedance-matching function* consists of three
mechanical advantages that dramatically increase the energy per unit
area at the fenestra vestibuli relative to the energy per unit area at the
tympanic membrane. The three factors are (1) the condensation effect
(or areal ratio), (2) the lever action of the malleus and incus, and (3) the
curved-membrane buckling mechanism of the tympanic membrane.
Together these factors are referred to as the **middle ear transformer.**

▼ **Middle ear transformer**
Impedance-matching func-
tions of the middle ear, consisting of the condensation
effect, lever action of the
malleus and incus, and
curved-membrane buck-
ling mechanism of the tympanic membrane.

Condensation Effect (Areal Ratio)

The effective area of the tympanic membrane (pars tensa) is approximately 17 times larger than that of the footplate of the stapes. Therefore,
sound transferred through the middle ear is collected over the relatively

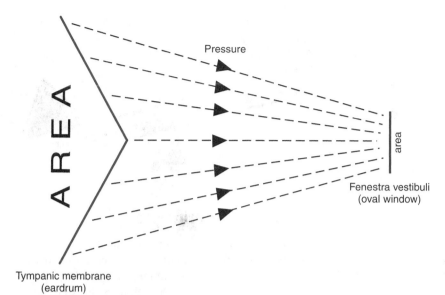

Pressure

AREA

area

Fenestra vestibuli
(oval window)

Tympanic membrane
(eardrum)

SIDE NOTES

FIG. 2-15
Condensation effect
(areal ratio).

large effective area of the tympanic membrane and applied to the relatively small area of the footplate of the stapes through the ossicular chain. Because pressure is equivalent to force/area, if force is held constant and area is reduced, there must be an increase in pressure. This is called the **condensation effect** (or **areal ratio**). The increase in sound pressure is equivalent to an approximately 24.6-dB improvement in auditory sensitivity (Figure 2-15).

▼ **Condensation effect**
Difference in area between the tympanic membrane and the footplate of the stapes, causing an increase in pressure.

Lever Action of Malleus and Incus

An example of a lever is demonstrated in a seesaw. If two children of equal weight are seated on a seesaw at equal distance from the *fulcrum* (pivot), neither will have an advantage in moving the seesaw. However, if the fulcrum is displaced so that one child is much closer than the other to the fulcrum, the one farthest away will have a distinct advantage. Figure 2-16 provides an example of this lever action.

In the middle ear the malleus and incus form a lever, with the manubrium of the malleus being 1.3 times the length of the long process of the incus, resulting in movement reduction from the malleus to the incus in a ratio of 1.3 to 1. This advantageous lever ratio results in sound amplification of approximately 2 dB as sound energy crosses the ossicular chain. This middle ear lever action helps offset the impedance mismatch between the air-filled middle ear cavity and the fluid (perilymph)–filled inner ear.

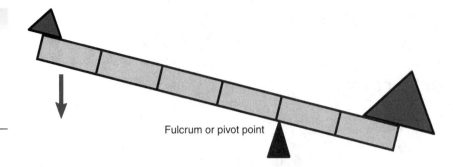

FIG. 2-16

Example of lever action.

Curved-Membrane Buckling Principle

Another contribution to the middle ear transformer action is made by the **curved-membrane buckling mechanism** of the tympanic membrane. This principle was described in the nineteenth century by the German scientist Hermann von Helmholtz. With the outside edge of the tympanic membrane firmly attached to the annulus and the membrane curving medially to attach to the manubrium of the malleus, the reaction to force is quite different in areas between the annulus and the manubrium than at the manubrium itself. As shown in Figure 2-17, a given change in force will result in greater displacement of the tympanic membrane than the manubrium of the malleus. The displacement is less at the manubrium, so the force will be greater; that is, the tympanic membrane itself acts as a lever, with the manubrium of the malleus as the fulcrum (pivot). Because the edges of the membrane are held firmly by the annulus, they cannot move, enabling the two portions of the tympanic membrane to act in a leverlike manner in force transfer (Figure 2-17). This mechanical action is estimated to increase force by a factor of two.

In summary, the transformer action of the middle ear provides approximately 32.9 dB of gain through the three mechanical advantages

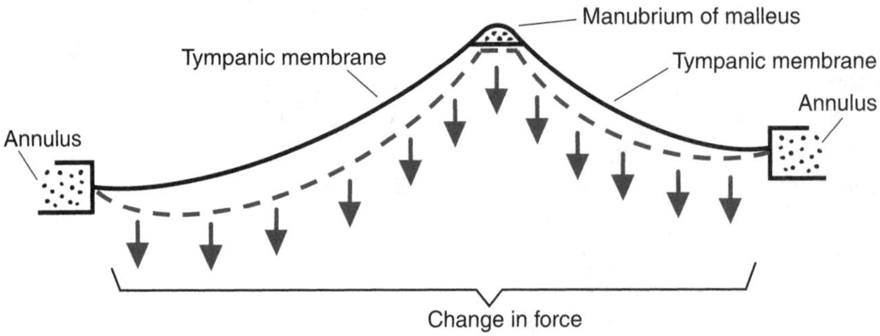

FIG. 2-17

Curved-membrane buckling principle. (From Tonndorf J, Kahanna SM: *Ann Otol Rhinol Laryngol* 79:743, 1970.)

Q & A
Question: How is 32.9 dB of gain for the transformer action of the middle ear derived? **Answer:** The summary calculation follows: 17 (areal ratio) × 1.3 (lever ratio) × 2 (tympanic membrane buckling ratio) = 44.2. To convert to decibel sound pressure level (dB SPL), we apply the following formula: $$20(\log 10_{10}\, 44.2) = 20(1.645) = 32.9 \text{ dB SPL}$$

described. This efficiently and effectively matches the impedance of air to that of the cochlear fluids.

These figures vary considerably among researchers. The effects also vary across frequency, making calculations difficult. Moreover, much of our knowledge of the transformer action of the middle ear comes from animal research, precluding direct application to the human system. Much inference and many mathematical models have been applied, which accounts for the differences in specific values seen in the literature.

Auditory (Eustachian) Tube

In order for the middle ear structures to function as described, the pressure on each side of the tympanic membrane must be equal. The primary function of the **auditory (eustachian) tube** is to ensure this pressure equalization. The tympanum is completely closed in by the tympanic membrane and bony cavity. The only opening to the outside environment is the auditory (eustachian) tube. This tube runs from a point approximately 3 mm above the anterior floor of the tympanum medially to the nasopharynx (see Figure 2-4). The *nasopharynx* is the area in the upper oral cavity and posterior nasal cavity. The nasopharyngeal opening (also referred to as the **ostium**) is normally closed, held in that position by the elasticity of cartilage and tissue surrounding the orifice and by the action of two muscles, the *salpingopalatinus* and *salpingopharyngeus*. The nasopharyngeal orifice opens each time we swallow, yawn, or sneeze by action of two muscles of the soft palate: the *levator veli palatini* and *tensor veli palatini*. Each time the nasopharyngeal orifice opens, air is allowed to move into and out of the tympanum, equalizing the pressure between the tympanum and the external environment *(atmospheric pressure)*.

▼ **Auditory (eustachian) tube** Tube connecting the middle ear cavity to the nasopharynx; its functions are to equalize air pressure on the lateral and medial sides of the tympanic membrane, provide the air supply needed for metabolism of the middle ear's tissues, and drain middle ear secretions into the nasopharynx.

Q & A

Question:
Why would the pressure in the tympanum be different than atmospheric pressure in the first place?

Answer:
The mucosal lining of the tympanum uses oxygen and nitrogen from the air (i.e., it consumes air). Without the pressure equalization function of the auditory tube, this consumption of air by the mucosa would create a negative pressure in the tympanum. In addition, atmospheric pressure is constantly changing, necessitating pressure equalization. The pressure changes we experience when flying or driving in hilly terrain produce pressure differences between the tympanum and the outside environment, with a subsequent "stuffy" feeling in our ears. Chewing gum, eating food, or any action that increases salivation and thereby swallowing often alleviates the problem.

▼ **Conductive hearing loss** Hearing loss resulting from impairment to any portion of the conductive auditory mechanism.

The auditory tube has three functions: (1) equalize air pressure on the lateral and medial sides of the tympanic membrane, (2) provide the air supply needed for metabolism of the middle ear's tissues, and (3) drain middle ear secretions into the nasopharynx. The auditory tube of a child is significantly shorter and straighter than an adult's tube. Moreover, children spend more time than adults in a reclining position, which reduces the efficiency of this tube, and they have a higher incidence of upper respiratory infections and allergic reactions. These factors result in children being more susceptible to middle ear problems than adults.

When any of these functions of the conductive auditory mechanism becomes impaired, from a myriad of factors, the resultant hearing loss is referred to as a **conductive hearing loss**. A problem in the conductive mechanism that interferes with the flow of sound energy from the outer ear through the middle ear (e.g., perforations of tympanic membrane, fluid in middle ear cavity) would cause a conductive hearing loss. Virtually any factor that may affect the function of the conductive mechanism is medically or surgically treatable. However, as discussed in Chapters 3 and 4, this is *not* the case with hearing loss resulting from loss of function in the inner ear or in the central mechanism.

ACTION OF MIDDLE EAR MUSCLES

▼ **Acoustic reflex** Contraction of the stapedius muscle in response to a loud sound.

As mentioned earlier, the **acoustic reflex** refers to the contraction of the stapedius muscle within the middle ear. This muscle contraction is bilateral (in both ears) regardless of which ear is actually stimulated, although the contraction is slightly stronger on the same side as the auditory stimulus (ipsilateral). The stapedius contracts at intensities of approximately 60 to 80 dB SPL (sound pressure level) when a noise stimulus is used to elicit the reflex (approximately 20 dB more if a pure-tone stimulus is used). When the stapedius contracts, the net result is to increase the stiffness of the system. Subsequently, low-frequency sounds are attenuated, with higher frequencies being relatively unaffected.

The tensor tympani muscle is known to contract concomitantly with increases in head and neck tension. As with the stapedius, the net result of the contraction of the tensor tympani is to increase the stiffness of the middle ear mechanism.

Contraction of the middle ear musculature has been found to attenuate sound by approximately 14 dB in the lower frequencies, but has little effect above 1000 Hz. This phenomenon, taken with the 60- to 120-msec latency (response time) of the acoustic reflex, would indicate that any protective function of the middle ear musculature is minimal.

Q & A

Question:
Why do we have the tensor tympani and stapedius muscles in the middle ear?

Answer:
The most widely accepted theory for the tensor tympani and stapedius being in the middle ear is that a contraction of these muscles will reduce hearing sensitivity for low-frequency sounds while not significantly affecting hearing for high-frequency auditory stimuli. This theory supposes that most sounds of life-sustaining importance in nature (e.g., eagle's screech, predator's breathing) are high-frequency sounds, whereas noise (e.g., wind in grass or trees, flowing brook) contains predominantly low-frequency sounds. Thus, it would be advantageous to us as well as to lower animals at present to reduce hearing selectively for interfering noise while still allowing the important high-frequency sounds to "come through" unaffected. Therefore, in this sense, contraction of these muscles makes the middle ear behave as a high-pass filter; that is, it passes high-frequency sounds while reducing the intensity level of low-frequency sounds.

SIDE NOTES

SUMMARY

The primary function of the conductive mechanism is to bring vibrational sound energy from outside the head to the inner ear for use by the sensory mechanism (i.e., to *conduct* sound wave energy to and through the outer and middle ear portions of the auditory mechanism). Sound wave energy passes into the auricle, then through the external auditory meatus, and strikes the tympanic membrane. The sound wave causes the tympanic membrane to vibrate, thus converting the acoustic energy from the sound wave into mechanical energy, through the movement of the tympanic membrane. This mechanical energy of the tympanic membrane is then transferred to the malleus (because of its attachment to the tympanic membrane), which in turn causes movement of the incus and stapes (because these three ossicles articulate with each other).

This anatomical arrangement of the tympanic membrane and malleus provides an efficient energy transfer and also serves to maintain the tympanic membrane's tense, cone shape. The malleus and incus act as a unit and vibrate in conjunction with the motion of the tympanic membrane. The incus passes energy along to the stapes (whose footplate is attached to the fenestra vestibuli). The stapes' footplate moves in and out as it is rocked by the incus, thereby transferring mechanical energy to the inner ear through the fenestra vestibuli.

The relative size of the tympanic membrane and footplate of the stapes, the relative length of the manubrium of the malleus and long process of the incus, and the curved-membrane buckling mechanism of the tympanic membrane provide the mechanical advantage necessary to match the impedance of air to that of the cochlear fluids. This transformer action provides approximately 32 dB of gain.

The middle ear contains the two smallest muscles in the body, the tensor tympani and stapedius. The stapedius muscle, innervated by cranial nerve VII, is responsible for the acoustic reflex. Both the tensor tympani and the stapedius increase the stiffness of the middle ear system when they contract, effectively producing a high-pass filter of incoming sound.

SUGGESTED READINGS

Durant JD, Lovrinic JH: *Bases of hearing science,* ed 3, Baltimore, 1995, Williams & Wilkins.

Seikel JA, King DW, Drumright DG: *Anatomy and physiology for speech, language, and hearing,* ed 3, San Diego, 2005, Singular Publishing Group.

Yost WA: *Fundamentals of hearing: an introduction,* ed 5, San Diego, 2006, Academic Press.

Zemlin WR: *Speech and hearing science: anatomy and physiology,* ed 4, Boston, 1998, Allyn & Bacon.

STUDY QUESTIONS

True-False

_____1.   The stapedius muscle is attached by means of a tendon to the neck of the stapes.

_____2.   The conductive mechanism of the human auditory system resides primarily in the outer ear.

_____3.   Damage to the outer ear or middle ear is permanent and not medically treatable.

_____4.   The middle ear is an impedance-matching mechanism.

_____5.   The footplate of the stapes rests in the fenestra rotunda (round window).

_____6.   The tympanic membrane consists of three layers of tissue.

Fill in the Blank

1.   The innermost (medial) ossicle in the middle ear is the _____.

2.   The orifice of the auditory (eustachian) tube that opens when we swallow, yawn, or sneeze is located in the _____.

3.   The instrument used to view the external auditory meatus and tympanic membrane is the _____.

Matching

Match the following terms (a-g) with the correct definitions (1-7).
a.   Annulus
b.   Tympanum
c.   Condensation effect (areal ratio)
d.   Auditory (eustachian) tube
e.   Cranial nerve VII (facial nerve)
f.   Lever ratio
g.   Cranial nerve V (trigeminal nerve)

1.   The tympanic membrane is approximately 17 times as large in area as the footplate of the stapes.

2. The manubrium of the malleus is approximately 1.3 times the length of the long process of the incus.

3. A connective tissue ring that retains the perimeter of the tympanic membrane.

4. Innervation of the stapedius muscle.

5. Middle ear cavity.

6. Pressure equalization function.

7. Innervation of the tensor tympani muscle.

Anatomy labeling

1. Landmarks of the auricle

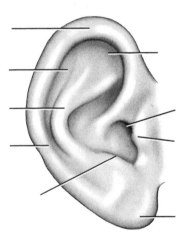

2.   Basic anatomy of the ear: outer, middle, and inner ear

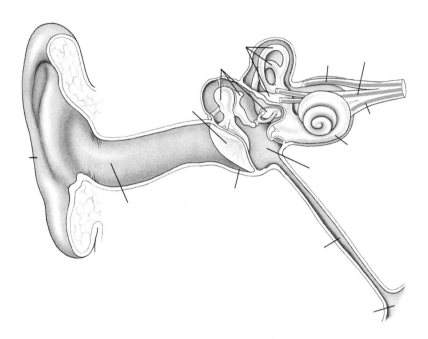

3.   Tympanic membrane

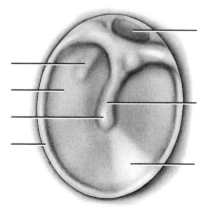

4. Middle ear

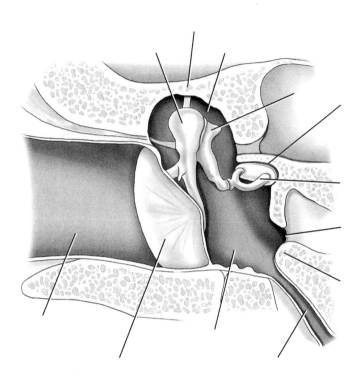

5. Ossicles

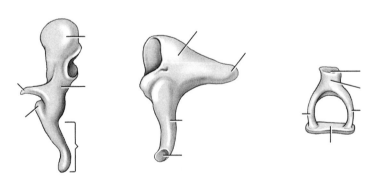

ANATOMY AND PHYSIOLOGY OF THE SENSORY AUDITORY MECHANISM

Inner Ear

Function of the Sensory Mechanism

Mechanical Properties
Active Processes
Cochlear Electrophysiology
Resting Potentials
Potentials Seen as Response to Stimulation
Single-Cell Electrical Activity

KEY TERMS

Labyrinth
Membranous labyrinth
Bony (osseous) labyrinth
Perilymph
Cochlea
Semicircular canals
Vestibule
Utricle
Saccule
Cochlear duct
Endolymph
Vestibular portion
Scala vestibuli
Scala media
Scala tympani
Reissner's membrane
Basilar membrane
Organ of Corti

SIDE NOTES

Stereocilia (cilia)
Cochlear nerve
Vestibular nerve
Statoacoustic nerve
Habenula perforata
Stria vascularis
Mass-stiffness gradient
Traveling wave
Spiral limbus
Depolarization
Otoacoustic emissions
Evoked otoacoustic emissions
Spontaneous otoacoustic emissions
Cochlear microphonic
Summating potential
Whole-nerve action potential
Tuning curve
Characteristic frequency

LEARNING OBJECTIVES

After studying this chapter, the student will be able to do the following:

1. Identify in detail the anatomy of the inner ear.
2. Describe the function of the cochlear and vestibular portions of the inner ear, and identify the major anatomical structures that comprise these portions.
3. Identify the three canals within the cochlea of the inner ear and the membranes that separate them.
4. Identify the branches of cranial nerve VIII that function within the inner ear.
5. Discuss the function of the hair cells in the inner ear.
6. Describe the transitional pathway of a sound wave through the inner ear structures, specifically the changes from mechanical to electrochemical energy.
7. Define otoacoustic emissions, differentiate evoked from spontaneous emissions, and discuss how they apply to the inner ear mechanism.
8. Discuss how the electrochemical makeup of the cochlea affects how sound is perceived.
9. Define endocochlear potential, cochlear microphonic, summating potential, and whole-nerve action potential.

10. Discuss the three responses to auditory stimulation that are attributed to the function of the cochlea.
11. Define tuning curves and discuss their derivation and role in our understanding of the auditory process.

Although the inner ear includes end organs for both vestibular and auditory functions, the discussion in this chapter is primarily limited to the auditory portion contained in the cochlea. The cochlea is very complex, with much still unknown concerning its physiological function. It is truly amazing that all information necessary to understand speech, appreciate music, or interpret sounds representing danger to the organism must be coded in this tiny structure, which is only approximately 35 mm in length. Information may be modified and refined in the central auditory system, but nothing can be added to auditory cues once the neurological signals leave the cochlea through cranial nerve VIII (statoacoustic nerve). With this in mind, let us look at this incredible structure.

INNER EAR

The inner ear is a fluid-filled series of canals that lie medial to the middle ear cavity in the petrous portion of the temporal bone. It is referred to as the labyrinth because of its mazelike arrangement. The labyrinth consists of two separate parts, with one part (the **membranous labyrinth**) contained within the other (the **bony [or osseous] labyrinth**). The bony labyrinth, the outer portion of the labyrinth, is filled with a fluid called **perilymph** and contains the **cochlea,** the three **semicircular canals,** and the **vestibule.** The cochlea and semicircular canals open into the vestibule on either end (Figure 3-1). The membranous labyrinth is composed of soft tissue and consists of a series of communicating sacs and ducts that conform to the shape of the larger bony labyrinth: the semicircular canals, **utricle, saccule,** and **cochlear duct** (Figure 3-2). It contains a fluid called **endolymph.**

The inner ear consists of two major functional parts: *vestibular* and *cochlear.* The **vestibular portion** is involved in the sense of balance and spatial orientation. It consists of three semicircular canals (*superior, lateral,* and *posterior*), each of which represents a body plane in space (see Figures 3-1 and 3-2). The canals are filled with a fluid that moves in conjunction with head and body activity. This fluid movement within the semicircular canals is registered in various parts of the brain that,

▼ **Labyrinth** Interconnecting, fluid-filled canals that form the inner ear.

▼ **Vestibular portion** Section of the inner ear that is involved in balance and spatial orientation.

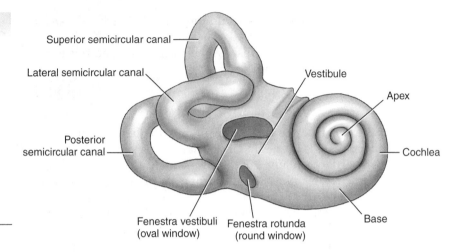

Superior semicircular canal

Lateral semicircular canal

Vestibule

Apex

Posterior semicircular canal

Cochlea

Fenestra vestibuli (oval window)

Fenestra rotunda (round window)

Base

FIG. 3-1

Bony labyrinth.

▼ **Cochlea** Section of the inner ear that is involved in hearing.

together with visual and somatosensory (muscle sense) cues, trigger appropriate muscle-motor actions to maintain proper body posture and stability with reference to the surrounding spatial environment.

That part of the inner ear mechanism involved in hearing is the snail shell–shaped **cochlea** (see Figure 3-1). The inner ear communicates with the middle ear through two small windows: the *fenestra vestibuli (oval window)*, which contains the footplate of the stapes of the ossicular chain, and the *fenestra rotunda (round window)*, which is located below the fenestra vestibuli and is covered with a thin, flexible membrane to allow for expansion as fluid movements occur within the cochlea (see Figure 3-1). The cochlea itself is a fluid-filled cavity. It is divided into three canals that extend its entire length from the base to the apex (Figure 3-3).

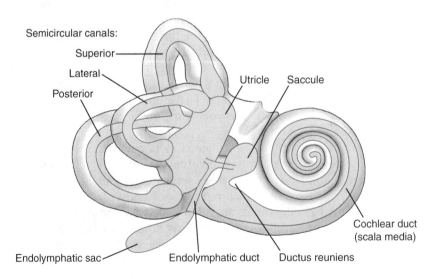

Semicircular canals:

Superior

Lateral

Posterior

Utricle   Saccule

Cochlear duct (scala media)

FIG. 3-2

Membranous labyrinth.   Endolymphatic sac   Endolymphatic duct   Ductus reuniens

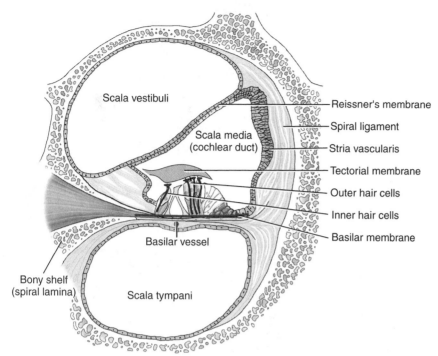

Scala vestibuli

Reissner's membrane

Spiral ligament

Scala media
(cochlear duct)

Stria vascularis

Tectorial membrane

Outer hair cells

Inner hair cells

Basilar membrane

Basilar vessel

Bony shelf
(spiral lamina)

Scala tympani

FIG. 3-3

Divisions of the cochlea
into the scala vestibuli,
scala media, and scala
tympani.

The **scala vestibuli** is one of the three canals; the middle canal is the **scala media** (also called the *cochlear duct*); and the **scala tympani** is the third canal. The canals are separated from each other by thin, membranous walls that allow fluid movement in one canal to influence fluid activity in the others. **Reissner's membrane** separates the scala vestibuli from the scala media, and the **basilar membrane** separates the scala media from the scala tympani. The scala vestibuli and scala tympani are part of the bony labyrinth, and the scala media is part of the membranous labyrinth.

The middle canal (scala media) houses the **organ of Corti**, the sensory end organ of hearing located on the basilar membrane (Figure 3-4). This membrane is approximately 35 mm in length. The organ of Corti consists of approximately 3500 tiny hair cells situated in one inner row and 13,500 hair cells in three to four outer rows from the base to the apex of the cochlea. These hair cells are the actual sensory receptor cells for the hearing process. The **stereocilia** (commonly called **cilia**) are small, hairlike projections on the tops of the inner and outer hair cells.

The basilar membrane itself is not uniform in width or thickness, but rather varies from narrow and thin at the base of the cochlea to wider and thicker toward the apex. This structural gradient results in mechanical differences related to the relative mass and stiffness of the membrane.

The **hair cells** of the organ of Corti synapse with the nerve fibers, which group together to form the **cochlear nerve,** a branch of cranial

▼ **Organ of Corti** Sensory end organ of hearing.

▼ **Hair cells** Sensory receptor cells for the hearing process.

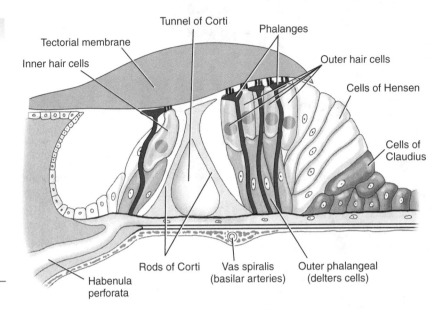

Tunnel of Corti

Phalanges

Tectorial membrane

Inner hair cells

Outer hair cells

Cells of Hensen

Cells of Claudius

Rods of Corti

Vas spiralis
(basilar arteries)

Outer phalangeal
(delters cells)

Habenula
perforata

FIG. 3-4

Organ of Corti.

nerve (CN) VIII. The **vestibular nerve,** another branch of CN VIII, originates from the semicircular canals and joins the cochlear nerve to form the statoacoustic nerve (CN VIII). The cochlear nerve sends nerve impulses from the inner ear to the cochlear nucleus in the brainstem (Figure 3-5).

The inner and outer hair cells differ in morphology. The outer hair cells are cylindrical in shape, whereas the inner hair cells are pear shaped. The arrangement of the cilia also differs. The cilia of the outer hair cells are arranged in a w pattern, with the top or open end of the w facing the tunnel of Corti and inner hair cells. The cilia of the inner hair cells are arranged in a shallow u pattern. Each outer hair cell has as many as 150 stereocilia, with approximately 50 to 70 on each inner

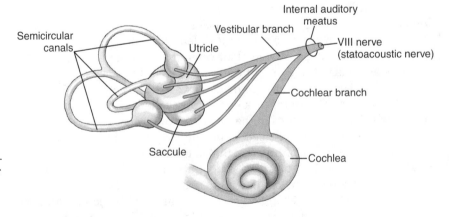

Semicircular
canals

Utricle

Vestibular branch

Internal auditory
meatus

VIII nerve
(statoacoustic nerve)

Cochlear branch

Saccule

Cochlea

FIG. 3-5

Cochlear and vestibular nerves are branches of cranial nerve VIII.

hair cell. The height of the stereocilia varies systematically from the base to the apex of the cochlea, with the shortest found at the base and longest at the apex.

There also are internal structural differences between inner and outer hair cells. Inner hair cells contain a chemical makeup that suggests a high metabolism, which may aid in transduction (conversion) of mechanical to electrochemical energy. The composition of outer hair cell cilia resembles muscle fibers, complete with contractile proteins in cell bodies and stereocilia, which enables them to change shape actively.

The *afferent* (ascending) neural innervation of the hair cells occurs through the cochlear branch of CN VIII **(statoacoustic nerve).** The inner hair cells are innervated by the inner radial fibers, which comprise approximately 90% of the afferent fibers. They enter the cochlea through tiny openings collectively referred to as the **habenula perforata** (see Figure 3-4) and course directly to the inner hair cells. Each inner hair cell receives approximately 20 radial fibers. The outer hair cells are innervated by the outer spiral fibers. These also enter the cochlea through the habenula perforata, then cross the tunnel of Corti and turn slightly toward the base of the cochlea before innervating the outer hair cells. Each of these fibers may innervate approximately 10 outer hair cells.

As mentioned above, approximately 90% of the afferent CN VIII primary fibers are innervated by *inner* hair cells; this finding is perplexing because very orderly correlations are consistently found between loss of sensitivity and *outer* hair cell damage. The outer hair cells may serve as an amplifier for basilar membrane displacement and facilitate inner hair cell activation. This at least partially explains the discrepancy. The auditory branch of CN VIII consists of about 31,500 nerve fibers and is only approximately 5 mm in length. It exits the bony labyrinth and enters the brainstem via the internal auditory meatus. At this point, it synapses with many other neurons in the cochlear nucleus at the junction of the pons and medulla.

In addition to the afferent innervation, both inner and outer hair cells receive *efferent* (descending) input. The efferent innervation is somewhat more extensive for outer hair cells than for inner hair cells. The fibers synapse directly with outer hair cells, but synapse only with the afferent neurons of the inner hair cells. These fibers descend from the superior olivary complex of the brainstem to the cochlea in the olivocochlear bundle. However, they receive input all the way from the cerebral cortex.

The cochlear blood supply is quite complex. The primary supplies are the **stria vascularis** (a vascular complex attached to the spiral ligament in the scala media [see Figure 3-3]) and a group of vessels just beneath the basilar membrane. The basilar membrane vessels appear to supply the organ of Corti with nutrients, whereas the stria vascularis maintains the chemical composition of the endolymph. There is no direct contact

SIDE NOTES

▼ **Stria vascularis** Vascular complex that maintains the chemical composition of the endolymph.

between the cochlear structures and the vascular systems, necessitating an intermediate transfer system, most probably the intracochlear fluids at each site.

FUNCTION OF THE SENSORY MECHANISM

The function of the cochlea is extremely complex. Mechanical, electrochemical, and active processes all contribute to transduction (conversion) from the mechanical movement of the conductive system components to the neural code that ultimately results in our detection and interpretation of the acoustic aspects of our environment. Despite centuries of inquiry, we still do not fully understand cochlear function.

Mechanical Properties

The sensory mechanism is a functional division of the auditory system that allows sound wave energy to be converted to neural impulses that are transmitted from the inner ear through the brainstem to the auditory cortex in the brain. As the footplate of the stapes moves within the oval window, the cochlear fluid develops corresponding increases and decreases in pressure (Figure 3-6).

The pressure changes result in displacement of the scala media because of the elastic membrane of the round window. That is, as pressure in the scala vestibuli increases from stapedial movement into the vestibule, this pressure results in displacement of the scala media toward the scala tympani. This movement results from the narrow junc-

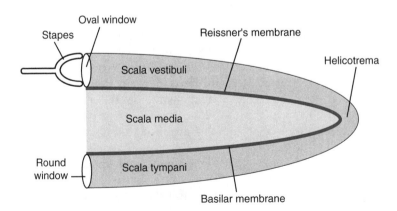

FIG. 3-6

An "unrolled" cochlea.

ture *(helicotrema)* between the scala vestibuli and scala tympani, which resists movement of perilymph through it, and from the elasticity of the round window membrane, which allows the fluid displacement. As the stapes moves outward, the elasticity of the round window membrane causes a pressure increase in the scala tympani relative to that in the scala vestibuli, resulting in displacement of the scala media toward the scala vestibuli. Displacement of the scala media includes movement of the basilar membrane, which, as we see later, causes the mechanical movement of the outer hair cell cilia.

At this point, we may summarize the sound pathway discussed so far. Airborne sound undergoes a number of transitions as it is processed through the auditory mechanism (Figure 3-7). Sound is airborne as it enters the external auditory meatus. However, once the sound strikes the tympanic membrane, its acoustic energy is converted to mechanical vibrations of the membrane itself and to the ossicular chain, which connects the tympanic membrane and the middle ear cavity located behind

Gross division	Outer ear	Middle ear	Inner ear	Central auditory nervous system
Anatomy	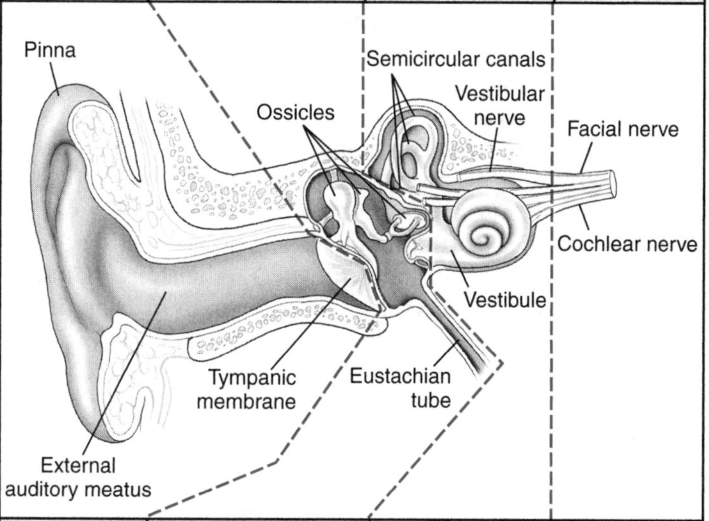			
Mode of operation	Air vibration	Mechanical vibration	Mechanical Hydrodynamic Electrochemical	Electrochemical
Function	Protection Amplification Localization	Impedance matching Selective oval window stimulation Pressure equalization	Filtering distribution Transduction	Information processing

FIG. 3-7

Diagram depicting the processing of airborne sound through the auditory mechanism.

SIDE NOTES

it. The ossicular vibrations are converted into fluid wave motions (hydrodynamic energy) in the cochlea, which houses the organ of Corti. The fluid wave motions cause the hair cells of the organ of Corti to be activated. In turn, the organ of Corti converts the fluid motions occurring within the cochlea into neural signals (electrochemical energy), which are transferred to the brain through CN VIII for final processing.

Recall that the basilar membrane varies in width and thickness from narrow and thin at the base to wider and thicker at the apex. In terms of mechanics, this results in stiffness dominating at the base and mass dominating toward the apex. This variation is called a **mass-stiffness gradient**. This gradient results in a change in resonance from higher frequencies in the stiffness-dominated portions near the base to lower frequencies toward the mass-dominated apex. The variations in resonance result in different frequencies of stimulation, causing maximum displacement of the basilar membrane at different places (i.e., the *resonant point* for each frequency).

If we look at the displacement of the basilar membrane for a pure-tone stimulus with frequencies of 300 Hz and 2000 Hz, we see disturbances that grow in magnitude from the base to the resonant point for the respective frequency, where it reaches a maximum. Figure 3-8 provides a schematic drawing of this phenomenon. Note that once the resonant point and resultant maximum displacement are reached, minimal disturbance of the basilar membrane occurs above this point (toward the apex). This complex pattern of vibration is referred to as the **traveling wave.** The displacement of the basilar membrane in response to stapedial movement is almost instantaneous across the entire length of the basilar membrane because of the high density of the cochlear fluids.

The point of maximum displacement is at a different place for different frequencies of stimulation. The displacement of the basilar membrane is limited by the attachment to the spiral lamina and spiral ligament (Figure 3-9). This arrangement results in a bending of the stereocilia of the outer hair cells. At least some of the outer hair cell stereocilia are in contact with the tectorial membrane; therefore, as the basilar

▼ **Mass-stiffness gradient** Difference in width and thickness from the base to the apex of the basilar membrane; results in variations in resonance and different frequencies of stimulation at different locations of the basilar membrane.

FIG. 3-8

Displacement of the basilar membrane in response to a pure tone shown at **A,** 300 Hz, and **B,** 2000 Hz. (From Zemlin WR: *Speech and hearing science: anatomy and physiology,* ed 4, Boston, 1998, Allyn & Bacon.

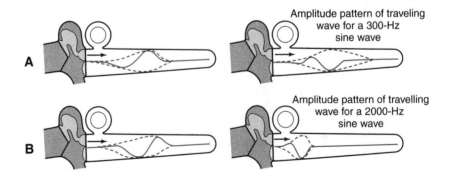

Amplitude pattern of traveling wave for a 300-Hz sine wave

Amplitude pattern of travelling wave for a 2000-Hz sine wave

membrane bows in the center, the stereocilia are displaced by their contact with the tectorial membrane (Figure 3-10).

The mechanical deformation then proceeds longitudinally along the basilar membrane from base to apex, with the displacement greater in the center than at the sides because of firm attachments at the spiral lamina and spiral ligament. This results in a bending or shearing of the outer hair

SIDE NOTES

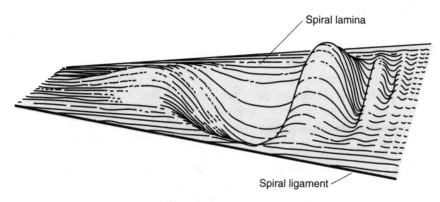

Spiral lamina

Spiral ligament

FIG. 3-9

Attachment of the spiral lamina and spiral ligament limits the displacement of the basilar membrane. (From Tonndorf J: *J Acoustic Soc Am,* 32:493, 1960, Acoustical Society of America.)

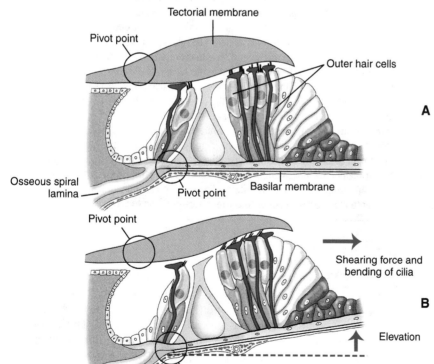

Tectorial membrane

Pivot point

Outer hair cells

A

Osseous spiral lamina

Pivot point

Basilar membrane

Pivot point

Shearing force and bending of cilia

B

Elevation

FIG. 3-10

Anatomical position of stereocilia in **A,** at rest, and **B,** in response to basilar membrane displacement.

cell stereocilia from contact with the tectorial membrane, which is firmly attached to the **spiral limbus.** Points of maximal displacement of the basilar membrane occur at different locations for each frequency component of a complex sound. This results in the basilar membrane performing a "mechanical spectral analysis" of each sound instantaneously.

Q & A

Question:
How do we move from mechanical to electrochemical changes?

Answer:
The details of hair cell activation are not fully understood. However, we can explore a feasible sequence of events that may result in initiation of a neural message. Tiny fibrous connections exist between cilia of the hair cells. These connections are called *links,* and they may be instrumental in neural activation of the hair cells and subsequent activation of the CN VIII nerve fibers.

On the inner hair cells, some of the links, called *tip links,* course from the body of stereocilia to the tip of adjacent stereocilia. Displacement of the basilar membrane toward the scala vestibuli (into the scala media) results in displacement of the cilia and subsequent stretching of these links, which can create an opening on the tip of the cilia through a "trapdoor" action. This opening allows for an ionic exchange that alters the electrical potential of the hair cell, which is called **depolarization.** The depolarization causes a neurotransmitter to be released at the synapse with innervating CN VIII fibers. this, in turn, eventually results in a neural discharge, which is part of the neural code representing a particular sound (Figures 3-11 and 3-12).

In applying this principle to the outer hair cells, the situation is not the same. It appears that the mechanical action is similar in the outer hair cells, but the result is a change in shape of the hair cell cilia (outer hair cell cilia resemble muscle fiber in composition). This change in shape or contraction and stretching may occur at the rate of the stimulus frequency, thus providing a boost to the basilar membrane movement at that point. In this manner, the outer hair cells may act as amplifiers of basilar membrane movement, with inner hair cells acting as the message-sending units. Approximately 95% of the afferent fibers synapse with inner hair cells. This long answer to the question leads us to active processes within the cochlea.

Active Processes

The previous discussion described contraction and change in the shape of outer hair cell stereocilia. This active response within the cochlea is a relatively recent finding. It has been known for some time that the cochlea produces sounds called otoacoustic emissions. These sounds may be in response to stimulation with clicks or carefully selected and arranged pure tones of very brief duration. These are called **evoked otoacoustic emissions.** Many people have otoacoustic emissions present without stimulation; these are referred to as **spontaneous otoacoustic**

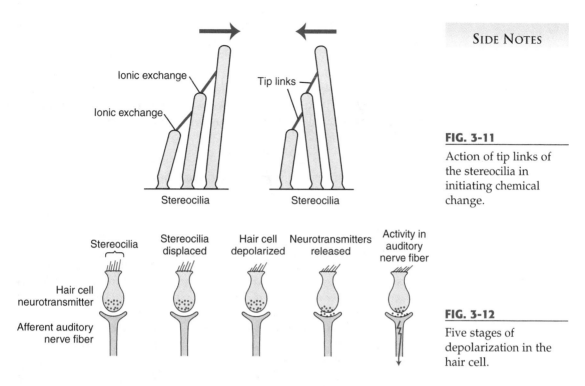

FIG. 3-11

Action of tip links of the stereocilia in initiating chemical change.

FIG. 3-12

Five stages of depolarization in the hair cell.

emissions. It is known that otoacoustic emissions are produced by the outer hair cells. Although a connection between the active shape alterations of cilia of the outer hair cells and otoacoustic emissions seems likely, it has not yet been confirmed empirically.

Otoacoustic emissions are used to screen hearing, particularly in neonatal populations and in audiologic diagnostics. It is likely that the measurement of otoacoustic emissions will be applied to clinical and research settings in many ways in the future.

Cochlear Electrophysiology

The electrochemical makeup of the cochlea appears to be the power supply that makes possible the initiation of the neural code that is ultimately perceived as sound. Many electrical gradients have been identified in the cochlea with and without stimulation.

Resting Potentials

Two primary direct current (DC) potentials can be measured in the cochlea with no stimulation necessary. The *endocochlear potential* is the

SIDE NOTES

largest of these, amounting to approximately +80 millivolts (mV). This potential, whose source is identified as the stria vascularis, is seen in the endolymph of the cochlea.

The hair cells have an intracellular resting potential of approximately −70 mV. This makes the potential difference across the top of the hair cells approximately 150 mV. That is, an endocochlear potential of +80 mV and an intracellular potential of −70 mV equals a potential difference of 150 mV.

Potentials Seen as Response to Stimulation

Potentials constituting a response to stimulation that can be seen in the cochlea include the cochlear microphonic, the summating potential, and the whole-nerve action potential (Figure 3-13). The **cochlear microphonic** is an alternating current (AC) potential that varies in exactly the same manner as the stimulus and is present only while the stimulus is present. This characteristic led some researchers to think that it was an artifact when it was first seen. The source of the cochlear microphonic appears to be at the top (cilia-bearing) end of the hair cells.

The **summating potential** is a stimulus-related DC response. It is a shift in the DC potential that can be either a positive or a negative voltage change and that is present only as long as the stimulus is present. As with the cochlear microphonic, the summating potential is a hair cell (i.e., receptor) potential.

As the name implies, the **whole-nerve action potential** originates not in the cochlea itself but in CN VIII. This response to a stimulus is only seen at the onset of an abrupt signal. The response represents a synchronized discharge of several CN VIII nerve fibers.

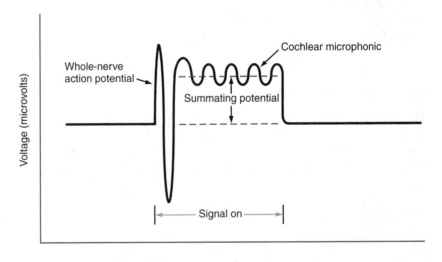

FIG. 3-13

Cochlear potentials in response to a brief, pure-tone signal with abrupt onset.

Single-Cell Electrical Activity

Using tiny wire electrodes insulated by glass or other nonconducting material, except for the very tip, it is possible to record the electrical activity of a single neuron. The electrode is called a *micropipet* and is moved as little as one micron (1 µm) at a time using a microdrive. This technique enables laboratories to isolate a single hair cell or neuron and observe its response to stimulation of the auditory system. The electrode is advanced until the spontaneous discharge of a target cell is detected by observing the electrical spikes representing discharges on an oscilloscope, then amplifying and routing them to a speaker, where they are transduced into an audible signal. Once the spontaneous discharges are clearly recorded, the spontaneous rate is noted, and changes in response to stimulation are observed.

One application of this procedure is basically to test the "hearing" response of the cell to various stimuli. As discussed in Chapter 5, the *audiogram* is a record of the lowest level of sound that an individual can hear and to which the person can respond at a number of different frequencies. When we look at the responsiveness of a single cell to a variety of frequencies, the record is called a **tuning curve**. The tuning curve may be considered an audiogram for a cell. To generate a tuning curve, stimuli of different frequencies are presented at increasingly high intensity levels until the discharge rate of the neuron increases. The level of the stimulus then is reduced to the lowest level that results in a

▼ **Tuning curve** Responsiveness of a single cell to a variety of frequencies.

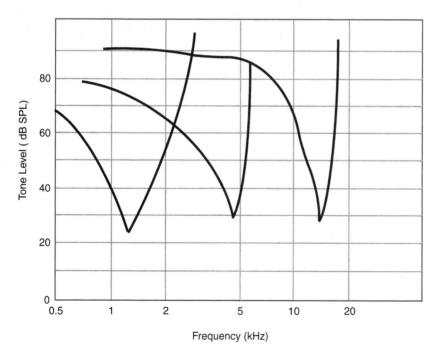

FIG. 3-14

Examples of tuning curves. *dB SPL*, Decibel sound pressure level; *kHz*, kilohertz. (Based on data of Kaing MYS, Moxon EC: *J Acoustic Soc Am* 55:620, 1974.)

detectable increase in firing rate above the spontaneous discharge rate. This is the neuron's *threshold* for that frequency. The frequency at which the lowest level of stimulation results in an increase in firing rate is called the **characteristic frequency** for that cell. This process is repeated at many different frequencies and recorded as a tuning curve. Figure 3-14 provides examples of tuning curves.

Recordings from individual cells have generated a tremendous amount of information about the auditory system. Complex experiments have shown the effect of many forms of stimulation on individual cells. When coupled with histological findings and data from other electrophysiological investigations, our knowledge of the auditory system is advancing rapidly, but there remain many mysteries to solve.

SUMMARY

The cochlea, through its mechanical structure and assisted by active response, analyzes sound and innervates neurons representing spectral and intensity characteristics of each component of that sound. Because of its minute size and inaccessible nature, the anatomical structure of the cochlea has been difficult to study. The structural variations in the cilia of hair cells, the mass-stiffness gradient, and the intricate arrangement of cilia and tip links all compose a mosaic that allows the cochlea to function. Neuron activation is caused by depolarization of hair cells, which occurs when displacement of cilia permits an ionic movement into the cell.

The neural discharge of cranial nerve VIII nerve fiber represents a code containing all the information available to the central auditory system to interpret the sound. However, much is still unknown about the function of the cochlea, and discrepancies exist between what is known from a physiological perspective and what is seen in psychoacoustic research, even as more is learned each day.

SUGGESTED READINGS

Durant JD, Lovrinic JH: *Bases of hearing science*, ed 3, Baltimore, 1995, Williams & Wilkins.

Greenberg S: Auditory processing of speech. In Lass NJ, editor: *Principles of experimental phonetics*, St Louis, 1996, Mosby.

Moller AR: *Hearing: its physiology and pathophysiology*, San Diego, 2000, Academic Press.

Tonndorf J: Dimensional analysis of cochlear models, *J Acoustic Soc Am*, 32:493, 1960, Acoustical Society of America.

Yost WA: *Fundamentals of hearing: an introduction*, ed 5, San Diego, 2006, Academic Press.

Zemlin WR: *Speech and hearing science: anatomy and physiology*, ed 4, Boston, 1998, Allyn & Bacon.

STUDY QUESTIONS

True-False

_____1. The bony labyrinth is filled with endolymph.

_____2. The cochlea is divided into three canals.

_____3. The basilar membrane separates the scala tympani from the scala vestibuli.

_____4. Inner hair cells contain fewer cilia than outer hair cells.

_____5. The organ of Corti receives nutrients from the stria vascularis.

_____6. The basilar membrane is wide and thick at the apex and narrow and thin at the base.

Fill in the Blank

1. The fluid-filled canals of the inner ear are called the _____.

2. The _____ contains the footplate of the stapes.

3. The two branches of cranial nerve VIII are the _____ and _____ branches.

4. The pattern of vibration of the basilar membrane is best described as a _____.

Matching

Match the following terms (a-g) with the definitions (1-7).
a. Hair cells
b. Tuning curve
c. Otoacoustic emissions
d. Stria vascularis
e. Habenula perforata
f. Perilymph
g. Organ of Corti

1. Sensory end organ of hearing.
2. Sensory receptors for hearing.
3. Openings in the cochlea for inner radial fibers of cranial nerve VIII.

4. Blood supply to the cochlea.
5. Fluid found in the osseous labyrinth.
6. Responsiveness of a neuron to a variety of frequencies.
7. Sounds produced by the cochlea.

Anatomy Labeling

1. Bony labyrinth

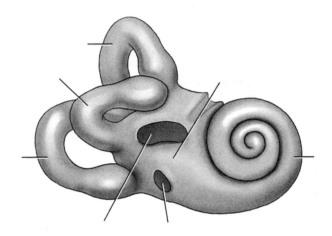

2. Membranous labyrinth

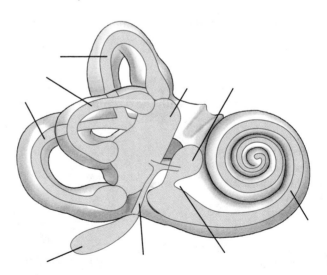

3. Cochlea

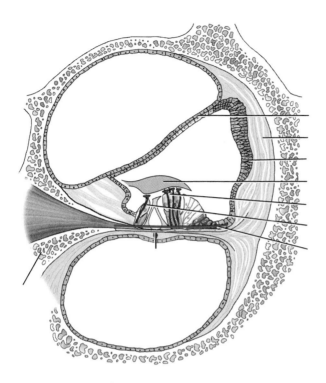

4. Organ of Corti cross section

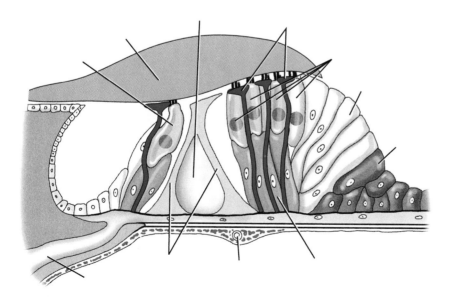

5. Branches of cranial nerve VIII

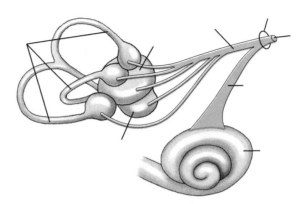

ANATOMY AND PHYSIOLOGY OF THE CENTRAL AUDITORY MECHANISM

Afferent Central Auditory Pathway

Efferent Central Auditory Pathway

KEY TERMS

Internal auditory meatus
Cochlear nucleus
Cerebellopontine angle
Diencephalon
Thalamus
Cerebral cortex
Longitudinal fissure
Superior olivary complex
Nucleus of lateral lemniscus
Response pattern
Internuncial neurons
Heschl's gyri
Lateral fissure (fissure of Sylvius)
Wernicke's area
Auditory cortex
Broca's area
Efferent auditory pathway
Centrifugal pathway
Olivocochlear bundle

LEARNING OBJECTIVES

After studying this chapter, the student will be able to do the following:

1. Identify the major elements of the central nervous system.
2. Recognize the different anatomical structures that make up both the afferent and the efferent central auditory pathways.
3. Describe the function of both the ipsilateral and the contralateral pathways.
4. Define response pattern and discuss it in terms of second-order and internuncial neurons.
5. Discuss the function of the superior olivary complex (SOC) within the central auditory system.
6. Identify the two functions that the inferior colliculus performs within the central auditory system.
7. Discuss the role of the auditory cortex and the superior gyrus in terms of sound, speech, and language production.
8. List the two primary functions of the olivocochlear bundle (OCB) and describe its role in the efferent auditory system.
9. Define the role of the centrifugal pathways in the efferent auditory system.
10. Describe the neurological pathway through which most auditory information travels to be processed.

As we have seen in previous chapters, airborne sound goes through many stages of change, resulting in a neural representation of the original physical properties. The mechanical movement of the middle ear structures, the hydraulic displacement of cochlear fluids, the movement of the basilar membrane intricately governed by static and dynamic mechanical components, and the active processes that amplify and refine the initiation of the neural code all occur almost instantaneously. The resultant neural representation of the original acoustic events may be modified only by reduction. As mentioned in Chapter 3, nothing can be added to information central to the cochlea.

The overall structure of the central auditory system is depicted schematically in Figure 4-1. Leaving the cochlea, cranial nerve (CN) VIII passes through the **internal auditory meatus.** This small channel through a part of the temporal bone also serves as a passage for a branch of CN VII (facial nerve) as well as the auditory and vestibular branches of CN VIII. Exiting the internal auditory meatus, the auditory branch of CN VIII courses a very short distance to the **cochlear nucleus,** the first major nucleus of the central auditory system, as shown in Figure 4-1. The cochlear nucleus is located at the junction of the pons and medulla

▼ **Internal auditory meatus**
Small channel through the temporal bone that serves as a passage for cranial nerves VII and VIII.

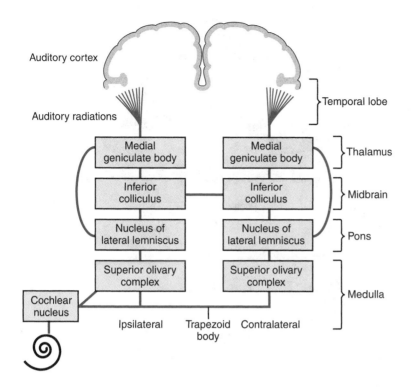

FIG. 4-1

Schematic of the structures that form the central auditory system. (From Deutsch LJ, Richards AM: *Elementary hearing science,* Boston, 1979, Allyn & Bacon.)

in the brainstem in an area referred to as the **cerebellopontine angle** (Figure 4-2).

We now look at the overall structure of the central nervous system as shown in Figure 4-2 to provide a frame of reference for our discussion. The brainstem lies superior to the spinal cord and, in ascending order, consists of the medulla, pons, and midbrain. The cerebellum, the coordination center, is located just superior and posterior to the pons and midbrain. The **diencephalon** lies just superior to the midbrain and contains the **thalamus,** which is a major distribution center for sensory activity. Above the midbrain is the **cerebral cortex,** which is composed of two hemispheres separated by the **longitudinal fissure.** Each cerebral hemisphere contains four lobes, or areas: the frontal, parietal, temporal, and occipital lobes (see Figure 4-2).

AFFERENT CENTRAL AUDITORY PATHWAY

The afferent fibers of CN VIII terminate at the **cochlear nucleus,** a major nucleus in the medulla that marks the beginning of the central auditory nervous system (see Figure 4-1). From the cochlear nucleus, there are

▼ **Cochlear nucleus** First major nucleus of the central auditory system, located at the junction of the pons and the medulla.

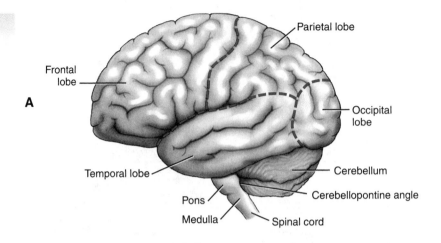

A

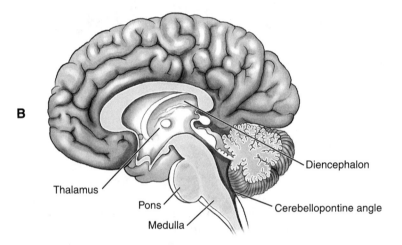

B

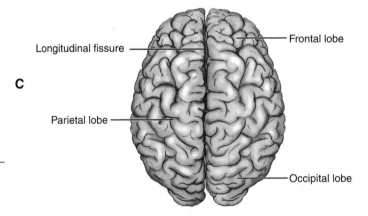

C

FIG. 4-2

The brain. **A,** Lateral view. **B,** Midsagittal view. **C,** Superior view.

two ascending pathways (or tracts): the *ipsilateral pathway* (the pathway on the same side of the brainstem as the stimulated cochlea) and the *contralateral pathway* (the pathway on the opposite side of the brainstem as the stimulated cochlea). Approximately two thirds of nerve fibers from the cochlear nucleus *decussate* (cross over) the brainstem between the cochlear nucleus and the **superior olivary complex** in the medulla, the next major nucleus. The neural tract that crosses the brainstem is called the *trapezoid body.* The remaining one third of nerve fibers ascend to the superior olivary complex on the ipsilateral side (see Figure 4-1).

Moving up the nerve pathway, the next major nucleus in the central auditory tract is the **nucleus of lateral lemniscus** in the pons region, followed by the **inferior colliculus** in the midbrain. The two inferior colliculi are connected by fibers that allow crossover from one side of the brainstem to the other side. Some fibers from the lateral lemniscus bypass the inferior colliculi and ascend directly to the next nucleus, the **medial geniculate body,** which is located in the thalamus. After this point, the afferent central auditory tract fans out into multiple small fibers called **auditory radiations,** which run from the medial geniculate body to the **auditory cortex** in the temporal lobe of the brain (see Figure 4-1).

The auditory reception area is located in the temporal lobe of each of the two hemispheres of the brain (see Figure 4-2). Perception of loudness and pitch (as well as many other simpler auditory behaviors) are controlled at the brainstem level, but higher-level behaviors (e.g., the understanding of speech and the processing of other complex signals) require normal functioning of the auditory cortex.

As discussed in Chapter 3, investigators are able to record from single neurons in the auditory system. In addition to determining the threshold of a neuron for various tonal stimuli (the tuning curve), the manner in which neurons respond to different auditory stimuli can be observed. Using a variety of stimuli, investigators can determine particular sounds and portions of sounds (e.g., onset or termination of the stimulus to which a neuron responds). Taken together, these single-unit results give us the **response pattern** of a neuron.

In obtaining the tuning curves discussed in Chapter 3, researchers observe the lowest level of stimulus that results in an increase in the firing rate of a neuron. However, to determine the response pattern of a neuron, a somewhat more complex analysis is needed. The firing rate of the neuron is recorded for very short intervals before, during, and after presentation of a stimulus. These recordings are averaged over many stimulus presentations, with the results showing the response pattern of that neuron.

Examples of different response patterns are shown in Figure 4-3. These graphs of firing-rate variations concomitant with stimulus presentation are called *post-stimulus time histograms.* They portray the manner

SIDE NOTES

▼ **Response pattern** Firing rate of a neuron in response to stimulation.

SIDE NOTES

in which the neuron responds to the stimulus (i.e., the response pattern). Every neuron discharges at some rate in the absence of any stimulation; this is called *spontaneous firing*. The rate at which the neuron discharges in the absence of any stimulation is called the *spontaneous discharge rate* and is indicated in Figure 4-3 as "spontaneous activity."

The cochlear nucleus may be divided into dorsal and ventral portions. The neurons that synapse with CN VIII fibers are called *second-order neurons*. Many of these neurons, particularly in the dorsal cochlear nucleus, have complex response patterns. Some respond only to the onset of a sound, whereas others respond only to changes in frequency, to the cessation of a sound, to complex bands of noise but not to pure tones, and so on. The manner in which many neurons in this area respond is also complex. Some increase the firing rate at the onset of a stimulus, then drop back to a spontaneous rate or below, and then increase again. Others show periodic increases in firing rate as long as

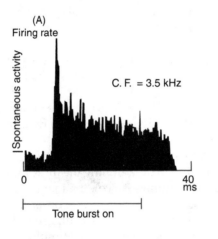

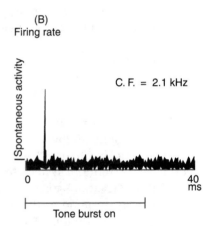

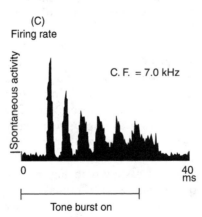

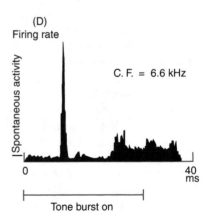

FIG. 4-3

Single-neuron firing patterns in the cochlear nucleus. *C.F.*, Characteristic frequency; *ms*, milliseconds.

a stimulus is present, whereas other neurons build in firing rate from a slight increase at the onset of a stimulus to a maximum as the stimulus continues.

Additionally, there are many **internuncial neurons** in the cochlear nucleus. These neurons are innervated by and innervate neurons within this nucleus. Many internuncial neurons may inhibit some neurons and excite others, introducing a level of complexity that defies description, and this is the most peripheral major nucleus in the central auditory system!

Most of the cochlear nucleus neurons with complex response patterns are located in the dorsal cochlear nucleus. On exiting this nucleus, many of these neurons ascend to the inferior colliculus, whereas neurons in the ventral cochlear nucleus project primarily to the next major nucleus, the superior olivary complex (see Figure 4-1). The majority of neurons in the central auditory system decussate, or cross over, to the opposite side of the brainstem at this point through neuronal bundles. As mentioned earlier, these bundles are called the *trapezoid bodies.*

The superior olivary complex (SOC) is the most peripheral point in the central auditory system to receive direct input from both cochlea (see Figure 4-1). The SOC controls the reflex activity of both middle ear muscles (tensor tympani and stapedius). When neurological impulses from intense sounds arrive at the SOC (through CN VIII), messages are sent down CN VII (facial nerve) to the stapedius muscle, causing a contraction of this muscle.

It appears that a primary function of the SOC is to code information necessary for auditory localization. Input from both ears is necessary for localization. The lateral nucleus of the SOC is sensitive to differences in the intensity of sound between the ears, whereas the medial nucleus of the SOC is sensitive to differences in the time of arrival of a sound between the ears. The information on time and intensity differences between the ears is the data primarily used to localize sound.

Q & A

Question:
Does the previous discussion mean that we could not localize sound sources if we were deaf in one ear?

Answer:
We could not effectively localize auditorily if we were deaf in one ear. This is slightly misleading, however, because we use more than auditory localization in locating and identifying a sound source (see chapter 5). In addition to audition, we use cognitive skills and experiential background in the localization process. For example, when a child who has no usable hearing in one ear hears a teacher call him, he does not become confused as to the source of the sound, but rather immediately turns in the direction where his experience tells him the teacher will be.

Returning to the auditory pathways, from the SOC, the primary central auditory tract ascends through the lateral lemnisci to the inferior colliculi. Some synapse at the nuclei of the lateral lemniscus, whereas others proceed directly to the inferior colliculus (see Figure 4-1).

The inferior colliculus is the site at which much of the information from the SOC is received. At this level, the information is synthesized and, in coordination with visual, vestibular, and somatosensory systems, results in a localization response. The *localization response* may be initiated at this subcortical level before cognizant awareness of the actions, as when we are startled by a loud or strange sound. Just above the inferior colliculus is the superior colliculus, which is a major site for visual localization. The proximity of these two major nuclei facilitates coordination of auditory and visual systems in localizing and identifying the source of any sound.

Localization is not the only function initiated at the inferior colliculus. The *startle reflex* also appears to originate here, with information relayed to the cerebellum and other higher centers. The neurological maze throughout the central system makes the most complex telephone systems in existence, complete with fiberoptics, appear simple.

From the inferior colliculus, the primary auditory path leads to the medial geniculate bodies of the thalamus. The thalamus is a sensory distribution center, routing information from the sensory systems to appropriate motor and higher sensory areas of the cerebral cortex and midbrain.

The coordination of the sensory systems and the motor system is essential; that is, it would do us no good to hear a train coming, localize it, and even to identify it, if we could not get out of its way. The medial geniculate bodies, inferior colliculus, and cerebellum are important in performing this coordination and distribution function. Much auditory information is directed to the *superior gyrus* of the temporal lobe through auditory radiations comprising **Heschl's gyri**. These radiations are located within the **lateral fissure (fissure of Sylvius)**. From here, information necessary for comprehension of speech is processed in **Wernicke's area** of the cerebral cortex, in the posterior portion of the primary auditory area (Figure 4-4).

The **auditory cortex** includes the superior gyrus of the temporal lobe and Wernicke's area on the posterior portion of the temporal lobe. There is little doubt that auditory information is processed in, and has an influence on, many other areas of the brain, but the auditory cortex appears to be the primary cortical site of processing auditory information. It appears that the left cerebral hemisphere is dominant in processing complex auditory information, including speech. This is proposed because lesions to the left hemisphere most often produce a language deficit (aphasia), the auditory cortex is physically larger on the left side than on the right side, and we show a right ear (represented in the left cerebral

▼ **Wernicke's area** Area of the left temporal lobe of the cerebral cortex that is important in the comprehension of speech.

▼ **Auditory cortex** Areas of the cerebral cortex that are the primary sites for processing of auditory information; these include the superior gyrus of the temporal lobe and Wernicke's area.

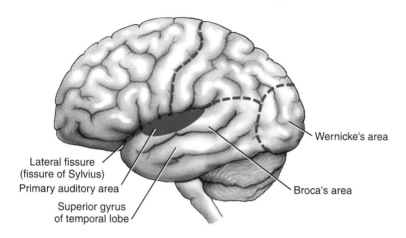

Wernicke's area

Lateral fissure
(fissure of Sylvius)
Primary auditory area

Superior gyrus
of temporal lobe

Broca's area

FIG. 4-4

Cortical auditory
reception area.

hemisphere) advantage in processing complex acoustic signals. At one point, cerebral dominance was thought to be a uniquely human trait. We now know that many birds, mice, monkeys, and other animals also show this phenomenon.

How we process speech and language is not completely understood. Results of extensive research and clinical observation suggest that much of the processing is done in Wernicke's area. Studies that monitor blood flow in the brain while subjects attend to speech have shown an increased blood flow in this area. These studies also have noted an increase in blood flow in **Broca's area**, or regions anterior to Wernicke's area that are thought to be involved in the production of speech.

In summary, it appears that the auditory cortex is involved in the processing of complex signals. Damage to this area interferes with complex signal processing, while often having no effect on more basic functions, such as auditory threshold and general localization ability.

▼ **Broca's area** Area on the inferior frontal gyrus of the cerebral cortex, important in the production of speech and language.

EFFERENT CENTRAL AUDITORY PATHWAY

The auditory pathway is primarily considered an *ascending* sensory pathway, but there is also a *descending* **efferent auditory pathway** of fibers, some of which originate in the temporal lobe of the brain and course all the way through the brainstem to the organ of Corti. The efferent auditory pathway is also referred to as the **centrifugal pathway**.

The **olivocochlear bundle** (OCB) is an important part of the descending efferent system; it descends from the SOC to the organ of Corti (Figure 4-5). The OCB has two primary components: the *crossed olivocochlear bundle* (COCB), which stimulates the contralateral cochlea,

▼ **Centrifugal pathway** (efferent auditory pathway) Auditory fibers that descend through the brainstem to the organ of Corti. The system is not well understood but is believed to provide an inhibitory function.

FIG. 4-5

Schematic depicting the relationship between the olivocochlear bundle (OCB) and the organ of Corti. *UOCB,* Uncrossed OCB; *COCB,* crossed OCB.

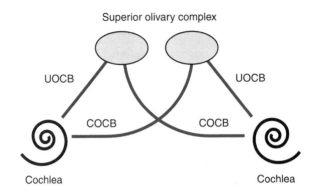

and the *uncrossed olivocochlear bundle* (UOCB), which stimulates the ipsilateral cochlea. The COCB affects primarily inner hair cells of the contralateral cochlea, whereas the UOCB affects primarily outer hair cells of the ipsilateral cochlea. Activation of either the COCB or the UOCB reduces the firing rate of CN VIII fibers responding to a stimulus or effectively worsens the threshold of these neurons for some auditory stimuli.

The efferent auditory system is not well understood. It provides an inhibitory function that can result in a significant increase in the intensity needed to initiate a response to a stimulus. Recall the potential mechanical amplification provided by the outer hair cells of the cochlea. This function may be inhibited by input through the OCB, thereby reducing cochlear output. Additionally, ample opportunity exists for inhibition throughout the central auditory system. There appears to be a constant "gating" of sensory input to the cerebral cortex, with information from one sensory system having priority at one instant and another a moment later. Even within the same system, we are able to emphasize one stimulus over another, separating figure from ground.

The role of the centrifugal pathways has received insufficient attention in the past. A primary function of this system is to prevent some afferent information from reaching higher centers. This system may account for how we can "tune out" sound while preoccupied with something nonauditory in nature, or allow certain sounds to come to consciousness while excluding others. When you are reading with the radio on, you often do not "hear" the radio; that is, you are not aware of it. If the radio mentioned your name or that of someone you know, however, you would suddenly be very aware of it. There is apparently a subliminal monitoring system that directs attention as a function of importance to the individual. This extremely complex system exemplifies the interaction of audition with the entire being.

Q & A

Question:
Is the efferent system affected by hearing loss?

Answer:
Activation of the efferent system depends on afferent input. Some of the afferent input is from other sensory systems, but some is also from the auditory system. Therefore, anything that affected the afferent input will affect the response of the efferent system. Many persons with hearing loss from cochlear damage complain of not being able to understand speech in the presence of background noise. This difficulty may be caused by a lack of efferent inhibition that aids in reducing noise while allowing signals to "come through." This view should lead to the understanding that cochlear damage not only results in a loss of auditory sensitivity, but also results in sensory overload. Viewing the problem from this perspective provides a much more accurate picture of the difficulties experienced by persons with cochlear damage.

SUMMARY

The central auditory system is much more than a conduit from the cochlea to the brain. The information leaving the cochlea is sorted, synthesized, and directed to appropriate portions of the central nervous system at each juncture. Actions such as the startle reflex, acoustic reflex, and localization responses are initiated at levels peripheral to the cerebral cortex, and complex analysis of speech, music, and multisensory construction of our environment take place within the cortex. Generally, complexity of function increases with progression from cranial nerve VIII to the cerebral cortex.

In addition to the information flow from the cochlea to higher centers, much neural energy flow also occurs from higher centers to lower areas, including the cochlea and the efferent system. Much of this neural activity is inhibitory or suppressive in nature. The efferent system appears to limit selectively the amount of information proceeding to the higher centers. This function reduces "sensory overload" and allows us to attend to sound or other sensory input that is of primary importance at a particular time.

The function of the central auditory system is not fully understood. We learn much from persons with impaired function of the central system (e.g., from cerebrovascular accident, head trauma, central processing disorders) as well as through laboratory research, but it will be some time before the complexity of the system is completely revealed.

SUGGESTED READINGS

Durant JD, Lovrinic JH: *Bases of hearing science,* ed 3, Baltimore, 1995, Williams & Wilkins.

Greenberg S: Auditory processing of speech. In Lass NJ, editor: *Principles of experimental phonetics,* St Louis, 1996, Mosby.

Moller AR: *Hearing: its physiology and pathophysiology,* San Diego, 2000, Academic Press.

Yost WA: *Fundamentals of hearing: an introduction,* ed 5, San Diego, 2006, Academic Press.

Zemlin WR: *Speech and hearing science: anatomy and physiology,* ed 4, Boston, 1997, Allyn & Bacon.

STUDY QUESTIONS

True-False

_____1. The first major nucleus in the central auditory system is the trapezoid body.

_____2. Fibers can cross from one side of the central nervous system to the other at the cochlear nucleus.

_____3. Most afferent cranial nerve VIII primary fibers are innervated by inner hair cells.

_____4. Perception of loudness and pitch takes place within the auditory cortex.

_____5. The localization response begins in the inferior colliculus.

Fill in the Blank

1. The first point in the central auditory system to receive input from both cochleas is the _____.

2. The _____ connect the medial geniculate body to the auditory cortex.

3. The medulla, pons, and midbrain are all parts of the _____.

4. Neurons that connect other neurons to each other are called _____ neurons.

Matching

Match the following anatomical areas *(a-f)* with the appropriate terms *(1-6)*.
a. Speech reception
b. Medulla
c. Speech production
d. Thalamus
e. Efferent auditory pathway
f. Midbrain

1. Medial geniculate body
2. Wernicke's area

3. Superior olivary complex
4. Inferior colliculus
5. Broca's area
6. Olivocochlear bundle

Anatomy Labeling

1. Lateral view of the brain

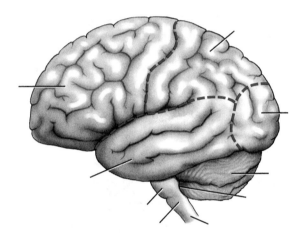

2. Midsagittal view of the brain

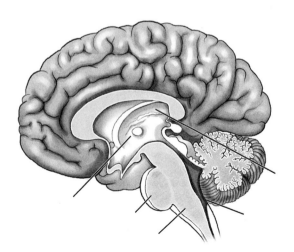

3. Superior view of the brain

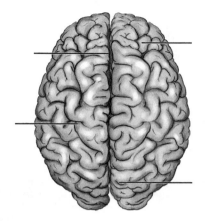

4. Cortical auditory reception area.

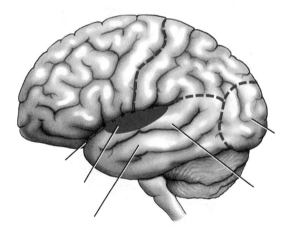

PSYCHO-
ACOUSTICS

NORMAL HEARING

Stimulus Characteristics

Stimulus Frequency
Stimulus Duration
Stimulus Intensity

Methods of Stimulus Presentation

Earphones
Speakers

Assessment of Auditory Sensitivity

Method of Limits
Method of Adjustment
Method of Constant Stimuli
Listener (Subject) Variables
Age Variation

What is "Normal Hearing"?

Localization of Sound

Intensity Cues
Time Cues for Localization
Hearing by Bone Conduction

KEY TERMS

Human audibility curve
Temporal integration (summation) function
Minimum audible pressure (MAP)
Sound field testing
Minimum audible field (MAF)

Reverberation
Incident sound
Reflected sound
Head shadow
Body baffle
Psychophysical methods
Tracking threshold
Two-alternative forced-choice procedure
Presbycusis
Sociocusis
Normal hearing
Audiogram
Head shadow effect
Azimuth
Lateralization
Minimum audible angle
Zero-degree azimuth
Bone conduction
Inertial bone conduction
Compressional bone conduction
Osseotympanic bone conduction
Occlusion effect

LEARNING OBJECTIVES

After studying this chapter, the student will be able to do the following:

1. Define threshold and identify the variables that affect minimum auditory sensitivity.
2. Identify the normal hearing range for humans.
3. Describe the effect of stimulus duration on auditory testing.
4. Define the auditory testing methods of minimum audible field (MAF) and minimum audible pressure (MAP), and describe how the variables inherent in each method differ.
5. Identify the three primary psychophysical methods used to determine threshold.
6. Describe the effects of age on hearing.
7. List the major factors that influence auditory threshold.
8. Assess and interpret the results of an audiogram.
9. Identify the primary cues used in auditory localization.
10. Describe the difference between hearing by air conduction and hearing by bone conduction, and list the three different subtypes of bone conduction hearing.

Normal hearing would seem to be a fairly straightforward, relatively simple topic. However, human hearing is more involved than it initially appears. Auditory sensitivity depends on many variables, including characteristics of the stimulus, method used in assessment, mental set and other listener variables, and method of stimulus presentation. This chapter discusses factors that influence sensitivity and introduces the application of these factors in a clinical setting.

STIMULUS CHARACTERISTICS

Stimulus Frequency

The human ear can detect an extremely wide range of frequencies. Although 20 to 20,000 Hz is often cited as the range of sensitivity, the lowest and highest frequencies in this range require sound levels that are quite high in order for them to be audible. We are most sensitive to frequencies from approximately 500 to 5000 Hz. The graphic representation of auditory sensitivity across frequencies is called the **human audibility curve** (Figure 5-1).

The area of most sensitive hearing contains most of the frequencies in speech signals. It may be fortunate in our society that we are not very sensitive to very low and very high frequencies. We are often exposed to sounds of 60 Hz from electrical appliances such as fluorescent lights that

FIG. 5-1

Normal human hearing. (Courtesy American National Standards Institute, 1969.)

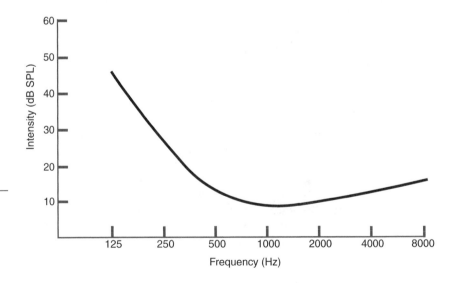

produce 60 decibels sound pressure level (dB SPL) and higher, as well as high-intensity sounds at 16 to 18 kilohertz (kHz) from various "ultrasonic" alarm systems. These sounds usually are not heard because of our poor sensitivity at these frequencies.

Stimulus Duration

The auditory system integrates energy over time up to a point. Our sensitivity improves as the duration of a stimulus is lengthened from the shortest duration that produces a perception of tonality—10 milliseconds (msec) for a wide range of pure tones—to about 300 msec. This change in sensitivity with duration is referred to as the **temporal integration (summation) function** (Figure 5-2). Sensitivity is not affected by lengthening signal duration beyond about 300 msec. As seen in Figure 5-2, the change in sensitivity for pure tones, as stimulus duration is lengthened from about 20 to 300 msec, is in the order of 10 dB.

The temporal integration function for persons with normal auditory function appears to be constant over a wide range of frequencies. Although some researchers have reported some frequency effects, careful examination of their subjects reveals evidence of some loss of sensitivity for higher frequencies, particularly 4000 Hz. We know that the magnitude of the temporal integration function is reduced for persons with hearing loss caused by cochlear damage.

▼ **Temporal integration (summation) function** A change in threshold as the duration of a stimulus changes.

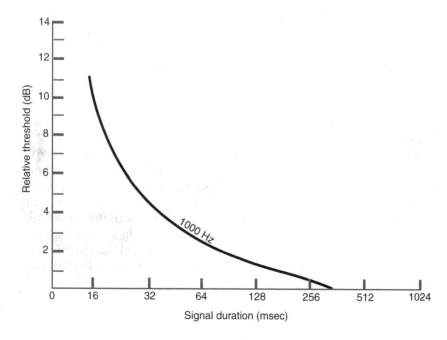

FIG. 5-2

Temporal integration (summation) function for persons with normal hearing. (From Deutsch LJ, Richards AM: *Elementary hearing science,* Boston, 1979, Allyn & Bacon.)

Stimulus Intensity

As previously discussed, we have a range of usable hearing regarding frequency. We also have a range of usable intensity. When a signal is barely audible, we must concentrate intensely to detect it. This concentration works well for a short time and sometimes enables us to identify the source of the sound, determine whether or not that source is threatening to us or otherwise of interest, and make a decision as to whether to ignore it, run from it, or chase it. However, if we had to concentrate that intensely over long periods, it would preclude doing much else. Therefore, sounds of very low intensity are usable and useful, but the utility is limited to relatively short periods. At the other extreme, sounds of very high intensity become uncomfortable (at approximately 100-110 dB SPL) and even painful. At levels of 130 to 140 dB SPL, we can actually feel the sound, usually as a tickling sensation. At these very high levels, most individuals will attempt to retreat from the sound as quickly as possible, so the usefulness is again short lived.

Despite these intensity-related limitations, the range of usable intensity is very large. If we define this range as extending from 10 dB below a comfortable listening level (approximately 40 dB SPL) to 10 dB below the uncomfortable loudness level (approximately 90 dB SPL), we have a 50-dB range of efficiently usable hearing.

METHODS OF STIMULUS PRESENTATION

Earphones

We typically present signals through earphones to make it easier to test right and left ears individually and to control the acoustical features of signals more accurately. When we measure auditory sensitivity with earphones, the result is called minimum audible pressure (MAP).

▼ **Minimum audible pressure (MAP)** Lowest level of sound heard when measuring auditory sensitivity through earphones.

Listening through earphones clearly is not a natural method. Use of earphones reduces the natural amplification afforded by the resonance of the outer ear, eliminates the slight increase in sensitivity from use of both ears simultaneously, and eliminates the effects of a reverberant acoustic environment. However, the increased ease of control of stimuli, isolation of ears, and reduction of ambient noise are major advantages of this method. It is important to keep in mind, however, that application of information obtained with earphones to hearing in everyday life must be done with caution.

Speakers

When stimuli are presented through speakers, it is called **sound field testing.** When sensitivity is assessed in this manner, the results are referred to as minimum audible field (MAF). When MAF and MAP results are compared, we find that MAF is more sensitive than MAP by 6 to 10 dB (Figure 5-3). The primary reasons for the increased sensitivity in a sound field compared with earphones appear to be the reduced contribution of the resonance of the external ear canal under earphones (see Chapter 1), the small increase gleaned from listening with both ears (binaural) in the sound field, and some technical variables related to calibration of earphones.

When listening in a sound field, there are several other contributing acoustic effects that are not prominent when listening under earphones. These include reverberation, head shadow, and body baffle. **Reverberation** is sound reflected from any surface. The sound coming directly from a speaker is referred to as **incident sound,** and that reflected from any surface is called **reflected sound.** Incident and reflected sound can interact, resulting in alterations of sound pressure level at various positions throughout the area. This variation in sound level caused by the interaction of incident and reflected sound is greatest for pure-tone stimuli, lessens for complex sounds, and is almost nonexistent for wide bands of noise.

Head shadow is a reduction of sound level at the ear on the far side of the sound source. This effect results from the head being between the sound source and the ear on the side away from the sound source (discussed later under Localization of Sound).

Body baffle refers to the acoustic effect of the body's presence in the sound field. The effect results from complex reflection and absorption

SIDE NOTES

▼ **Minimum audible field (MAF)** Lowest level of sound heard when stimuli are presented through speakers.

▼ **Head shadow** Reduction of sound level at the ear farther away from the sound source, caused by the presence of the head between the sound source and the ear.

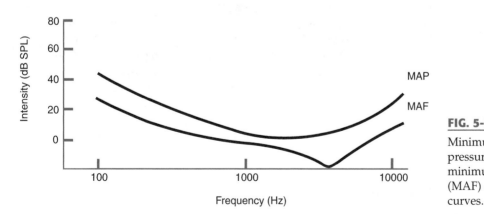

FIG. 5-3

Minimum audible pressure (MAP) and minimum audible field (MAF) audibility curves.

of sound by the physical presence of the body. This effect will vary depending on the type of clothing worn and body size.

ASSESSMENT OF AUDITORY SENSITIVITY

The manner in which we assess auditory sensitivity has an influence on the results obtained. The methods applied in determining sensitivity are called **psychophysical methods.** As the name implies, psychophysical methods are a means of coupling physical properties of a stimulus to the perception of and response to that stimulus. It is important to keep in mind that we normally determine when a person detects a stimulus by asking the individual to indicate in some way that he or she has detected it. That is, the physical stimulus is processed through the psychological as well as physical characteristics of the subject before the observable response occurs.

Three psychophysical methods that link the stimulus to a response are the method of limits, method of adjustment, and method of constant stimuli.

Method of Limits

Application of the method of limits entails changing one parameter of the auditory stimulus, in this case *intensity,* by the person performing the assessment (examiner), with the person being tested (subject) asked to indicate in some way when he or she detects the stimulus. The subject may be asked to raise a hand, push a button, or use any other behavior that is observable to the examiner, each time the subject hears the stimulus. The examiner may initially present the stimulus at a level that is clearly audible to the subject, then decrease intensity between presentations until it is inaudible (*descending* approach). Alternatively, the examiner may initially present the stimulus at a very low level that is inaudible to the subject, then increase intensity between presentations until it is audible (*ascending* approach). Thresholds obtained using a descending approach are generally 3 to 4 dB more sensitive than those obtained using an ascending approach.

Method of Adjustment

The method of adjustment involves having the subject adjust some parameters, in this case the intensity level of the stimulus, to a point where it is barely audible. Variations in this method include employing special equipment that varies frequency slowly as the subject controls the intensity. The subject is asked to keep the signal barely audible by using a button that controls the intensity. The subject's variations of stimulus intensity are recorded, resulting in a record of sensitivity across frequencies. This is called the **tracking threshold.** Threshold obtained using this method varies depending on exactly where on the recorded excursions the examiner marks threshold.

Method of Constant Stimuli

The method of constant stimuli uses a technique called the **two-alternative forced-choice procedure.** To apply this technique, an approximation of sensitivity for a particular stimulus is made using the method of limits or the method of adjustment. Several levels (e.g., 1 dB or 0.5 dB apart) above and below this approximation are then selected. Each of these levels is presented up to 100 times in random order. Usually, no stimulus is presented in some periods, randomly interspersed with the various levels of stimulus. The subject then is asked to indicate "yes" or "no" during each period when a stimulus may be presented. These time periods are indicated by a visual cue such as a light. A "yes" response indicates that the listener detected a stimulus, and a "no" indicates that no stimulus was detected.

When testing is completed, results are plotted as to the percentage of time each level of stimulus was detected (i.e., what percentage of time each level received a "yes" response during the period that it was presented). Some percentage of correct responses is determined to constitute the individual's *threshold.* Figure 5-4 shows the results obtained using the method of constant stimuli, with a 50% response level defined as the threshold.

This discussion of the method of constant stimuli raises questions about what threshold is. Within limits, "threshold" is whatever operational definition the examiner indicates. In Figure 5-4 the operational definition is given as the 50% correct response level, which yields a value of 15 dB SPL. If the operational definition were changed to 100% correct response level, the threshold value would be 18 dB SPL; at 30% correct response level the value would be 13.5 dB SPL; and so on. Threshold is a measure of sensitivity. It is not a static value, but rather a dynamic metric with variations dependent upon many factors, as discussed previously or later.

Listener (Subject) Variables

Subjects vary in their predisposition to determine whether a stimulus is heard or not. That is, some persons are predisposed to respond if they

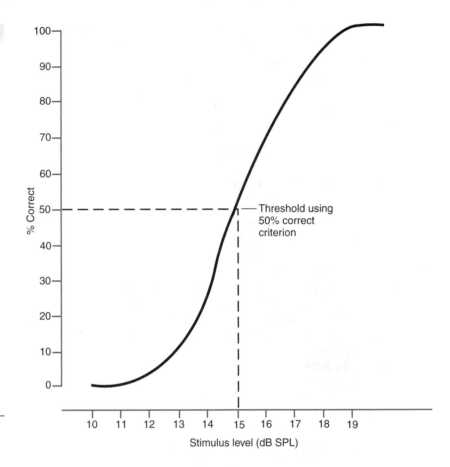

FIG. 5-4

Method of constant stimuli.

even think that they hear something while being tested, whereas others wait until a signal is clearly audible before acknowledging its presence. This predisposition, or *preparatory set,* can be altered to a considerable extent by the directions given by the examiner. An example is an individual found to respond frequently when no stimulus is being presented; this is called a *false-positive* response. The examiner might instruct this person only to respond when he is certain that he hears the stimulus. Conversely, if a subject waits until the stimulus is well above threshold before responding,* she may be instructed to respond when she even thinks that she hears the stimulus.

---

*This is often indicated by the subject cocking the head or by changes in facial expression concomitant with a stimulus presentation.

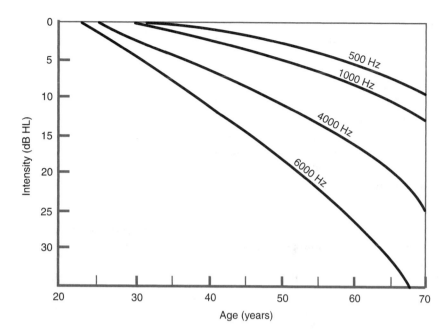

SIDE NOTES

FIG. 5-5

Auditory threshold as a function of age. *HL,* Hearing level. (From Deutsch LJ, Richards AM: *Elementary hearing science,* Boston, 1979, Allyn & Bacon.)

Age Variation

At least in our society, persons usually begin to lose hearing sensitivity at approximately 25 to 30 years of age. The loss of hearing begins in the higher frequencies (3000-6000 Hz) and worsens in degree of loss and range of frequencies affected throughout life (Figure 5-5). This loss of hearing is found to be greater in men than in women. This age-related loss of hearing was initially called **presbycusis** and was thought to be caused by the aging process. However, we now know that in some societies this deterioration of hearing with age does not occur to a significant extent, which tends to indicate that aging alone is not the cause. Possible societal factors include noise and dietary differences. Many persons now refer to this progressive hearing loss as socioacusis.

Regardless of the term used, we do lose hearing as we age, and this loss is increased by exposure to high levels of noise. However, whether the cause is aging, noise, dietary considerations, or other factors, or a combination, is not known at this time.

▼ **Socioacusis (presbycusis)** Hearing loss usually associated with the aging process.

WHAT IS "NORMAL HEARING"?

With all the contributors to variability in auditory threshold previously discussed, one might wonder if there is really such a thing as normal hearing. **Normal hearing** sometimes seems to be one of those concepts that everyone thinks they know but that no one can define satisfactorily. This section discusses some perspectives and issues concerning normal hearing.

Persons first became interested in quantifying hearing sensitivity in the 1930s. The primary impetus for this early work was communication, and extensive research was conducted in the Bell Telephone Laboratories. In the 1940s, diagnostic and aural rehabilitation perspectives were added. It became evident early that determining threshold in dB SPL could be cumbersome and confusing. Recall that hearing sensitivity varies across frequency. This means that in dB SPL, normal hearing, and subsequently hearing loss, would need to be defined differently at each frequency.

To simplify this problem, various organizations over the years consolidated large amounts of data on hearing threshold at many frequencies for young adults with no auditory pathology (i.e., "normals"). They then took the median threshold of this huge number of persons and made it "zero" decibel hearing level (dB HL). This is the zero reference we use in testing hearing in a clinical setting. The organization presently stipulating standards for audiometric assessment is the American National Standards Institute (ANSI). ANSI publishes the norms for audiometric zero for each frequency and delineates how it is to be determined. To calibrate to ANSI standards, we must measure the output of earphones in a 6-mL coupler. Six milliliters has been determined to be the approximate volume under commonly used earphones, including the external auditory canal and concha in adults.

Another factor that had to be determined early was what frequencies to test. It was known that physiologically equal distances along the basilar membrane separated points most responsive to frequencies one octave apart. Thus, from a diagnostic point of view, it made sense to test in octave steps to "sample" equal distances along the basilar membrane. Since these early years, we have learned the value of threshold measurements at several intraoctave frequencies in addition to octave steps. Generally, we test hearing at 250, 500, 1000, 2000, 3000, 4000, 6000, and 8000 Hz, and in some cases we test at 750 and 1500 Hz, as well as frequencies much greater than 8000 Hz. The record of thresholds at these frequencies is called an **audiogram** (Figure 5-6).

▼ **Audiogram** Graph or table showing thresholds in hearing level at different frequencies.

Remember that threshold depends partly on the operational definition of the examiner. In clinical audiology, *threshold* is defined as the lowest level of stimulus that the subject, or patient, responds to at least two out of three times.

Once we obtain an audiogram, we must use it to make judgments about several issues, such as separating normal from abnormal sensitivity. Despite approximately 65 years of audiometric assessments, there

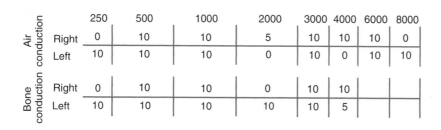

		250	500	1000	2000	3000	4000	6000	8000
Air conduction	Right	0	10	10	5	10	10	10	0
	Left	10	10	10	0	10	0	10	10
Bone conduction	Right	0	10	10	0	10	10		
	Left	10	10	10	10	10	5		

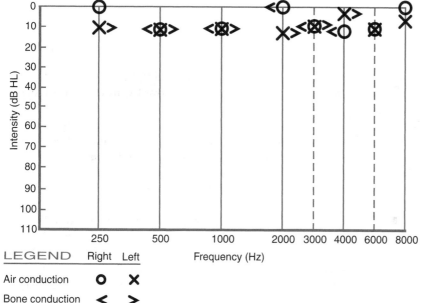

LEGEND   Right Left   Frequency (Hz)

	Right	Left
Air conduction	O	X
Bone conduction	<	>

FIG. 5-6

Numerical (top) and graphic (bottom) audiograms for a person with normal hearing.

is no universally accepted criterion of what is "normal." This partly results from a need to assess and evaluate each audiogram within the framework of all aspects of the individual. In addition, opinions differ as to what level of hearing represents the onset of difficulty in day-to-day life. Some believe that a threshold of 25 dB HL or higher across frequencies is normal, and that less sensitive hearing constitutes a problem. Others think that 20 dB HL is a more appropriate cutoff; others believe that any definition should be frequency specific (i.e., not include some high frequencies); and still others advocate a standard that varies with age because all of us will lose some sensitivity with aging. Again, although everyone seems to know what normal hearing is, no universal definition exists.

LOCALIZATION OF SOUND

Normally, the primary cues used in auditory localization are time and intensity differences between the ears. Chapter 4 discusses the role of the central auditory system in this process. This section focuses on the acoustic aspects that create the differences between ears.

Intensity Cues

When the source of a sound is not directly in front of or behind us, there is a difference in the intensity of the sound between the ears. This difference results partially from the difference in distance (i.e., one ear will be closer to the sound source) and, more importantly, from the obstruction provided by the head itself (head shadow). Recall that when a sound encounters an object larger than its wavelength, it is reflected or absorbed by that object. This results in the sound being considerably more intense on the side toward the sound source (the *near side*) than on the side away from the sound source (the *far side*). For any given object, this effect will be greatest for higher frequencies (i.e., shorter wavelengths).

The **head shadow effect** usually is greatest when the sound comes from the side of the head, but it is also a significant factor when the sound arrives at smaller angles to the head. The angle of incidence of the sound is referred to as the **azimuth.** A zero-degree (0°) azimuth indicates that the sound source is directly in front of the listener; a 90-degree (90°) azimuth means that the sound source is directly to the right; and a 180-degree (180°) azimuth shows that the sound source is directly behind the listener. The head shadow effect is much more important in causing an interaural difference than the relatively small intensity loss that occurs because of the distance between near and far ear, although these effects are additive. The central auditory system interprets the interaural intensity difference as sound coming from the side receiving the greater intensity.

The azimuth of the sound source also affects the resonance of the external auditory canal. This effect, coupled with head shadow, results in dramatic changes in the intensity of a sound between the ears as the azimuth changes. This is evident if we observe a dog or cat localizing the source of an interesting sound. If the source is not visible on turning in the general direction of the source, the animal will move or "cock" his head trying to narrow the field to search visually.

The head shadow effect and canal resonance effect are greatest at higher frequencies, so the interaural intensity difference cue is large enough to allow for the localization of tones of approximately 2000 Hz

▼ **Azimuth** Angle of incidence of a sound wave as it reaches the head. A zero-degree azimuth indicates that the sound is directly in front of the head.

and higher (wavelength = velocity/frequency; 2000-Hz wavelength = 1130 ft per sec/2000 Hz = 0.56 ft, or 6.7 inches). This effect can be demonstrated under somewhat artificial conditions. If an identical pure tone is presented simultaneously to both ears under headphones, the listener will say that the tone is coming from somewhere in the middle of the head. If the tone in the right ear were increased in intensity relative to the one in the left ear, the listener would perceive the sound source as moving to the right. This phenomenon is referred to as **lateralization.** When the difference between the intensity of the tones reaches approximately 30 to 40 dB, the listener would be unaware that the tone of lesser intensity were even present; that is, the listener would hear the tone in the right ear and be unaware of the tone in the left ear.

Time Cues for Localization

Interaural intensity differences most effectively account for the localization of tones at higher frequencies, and we know that we can localize tones of all frequencies. Therefore, another cue must account for the localization of tones of lower frequencies.

The speed of sound (velocity) is constant within a medium, traveling about 1130 feet (340 meters, 34,000 cm) per second in the medium of air regardless of the sound's frequency. The distance that sound must travel is greater to the *far ear* than to the *near ear* for both 45-degree and 90-degree conditions, but the difference is somewhat greater for a 90-degree azimuth. Translated into time, a tone directed at a 45-degree angle to the head will arrive at the near ear approximately 0.4 msec sooner than to the far ear, and the difference will be approximately 0.65 msec if the azimuth is 90 degrees (Figure 5-7).

In a laboratory environment, using earphones, interaural time differences as small as 10 microseconds (millionths of a second, μsec) have produced *lateralization effects,* that is, perceptions of the sound localized to the ear receiving the signal sooner than the other ear.

Localization using time as a cue is not limited to the time of arrival at the two ears, but also uses the difference in phase of component pure tones between ears. For lower frequencies, the wavelength of pure tones exceeds the approximate 7 inches between the ears. This results in a difference in the phase of the signal between the ears at frequencies below approximately 1800 Hz. Recall that hair cells in the cochlea are phase sensitive, often depolarizing in response only to the rarefaction phase of a pure tone. These phase differences may serve as a localization cue for lower-frequency components of sound.

As with intensity cues, both absolute time of arrival and phase differences are not isolated, passive events but are enhanced by head movement and subsequent coordination with somatosensory information.

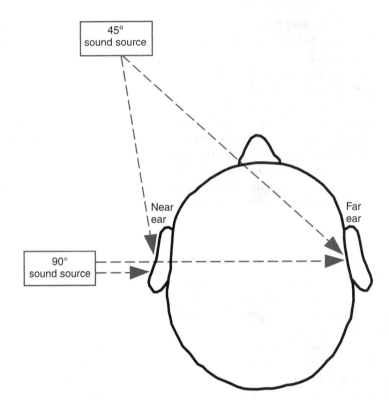

FIG. 5-7

Distance/time of sound
to the near and far ears
from two different
angles.

▼ **Minimum audible angle**
Smallest separation of angles
of incidence that can be
perceived.

Thus, the auditory system does not operate alone, but rather is an integral part of the total organism.

Our ability to localize sound is excellent. The ability to tell when a sound has changed position is measured or expressed in terms of the **minimum audible angle,** which is the smallest angular separation that can be perceived. The minimum audible angle varies, depending on the direction from which the sound is coming relative to head position. That is, when we are oriented directly toward the sound source, looking straight at it (called the **zero-degree azimuth**), we can detect very small changes in the lateral position of the source. However, a sound source beginning at 90 degrees (straight to our right), 270 degrees (straight to our left), or 180 degrees (directly behind us) must be moved a much greater distance before we can perceive that it has moved.

Keeping in mind that a primary function of the auditory system is to direct the visual, tactile, and olfactory senses in an effort to identify components of our environment, this localization makes sense. For example, if a sound is suddenly heard to the listener's left, the auditory system, coordinating with the entire central nervous system, will direct a turn to the left; the visual system will sweep that area in an attempt to identify the source of that sound. If the source of the sound is not identified readily by the visual system, the auditory system will use the smaller minimum audible angle at or near the zero-degree azimuth to narrow the area on which the visual system will focus. This process will continue until the source of the sound is identified. At the same time, all other sensory systems will be "placed on alert" until the sound source is identified and a decision is made to explore it further or to avoid it.

In summary, research supports a predominantly two-factor system in accounting for the localization of pure tones, with *time* cues serving as the important cues for the localization of lower frequencies and *intensity* cues serving the localization of higher frequencies. Because most sounds that we hear in nonlaboratory situations (including speech, noise, and music) are complex signals that contain both low-frequency and high-frequency components, both interaural intensity difference and interaural time difference are cues used by the auditory system when it makes localization judgments of complex sounds.

It is important to remember that the auditory system does not exist in isolation, but rather is one part of a very complex whole. When a child is seen with a profound hearing loss in one ear, it is often anticipated that the child will be unable to localize sound sources. Although it is true that auditory localization is minimal with only one usable ear, we use much more than auditory cues to localize a sound source. Children with no usable hearing in one ear usually will still turn toward the parent or teacher calling them because they know where that person normally is located. When we are standing beside a building and hear aircraft sounds, we look up even though reverberation often precludes our use of auditory localization cues. These are examples of the use of experiential background in our localization efforts. Again, the auditory system is only one part of the entire organism. Thus, it cooperates with visual, olfactory, tactile, and cognitive systems in defining and interpreting our environment. This interaction of sensory systems also allows us to move our heads in localizing, enabling a complex analysis of the effect of head movement on interaural time and intensity differences.

Hearing by Bone Conduction

Thus far we have talked about hearing through the most common mode: airborne sound received by the outer and middle ears, activating the cochlea. Another mode of stimulation of the cochlea is by setting the bones of the skull into vibration (Figure 5-8).

The stimulation at the cochlear level is the same regardless of which mode of stimulation is used. If we strike a tuning fork, we can hear the resultant pure tone by air conduction. If we put earplugs in both ears and strike the tuning fork again, we may hear it at first, but it will

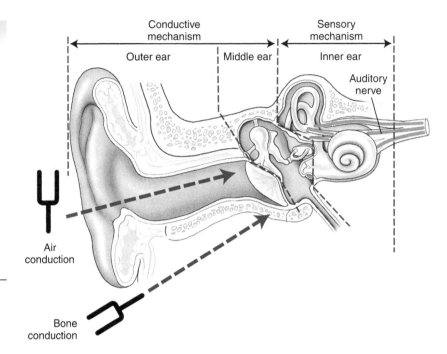

Conductive mechanism

Sensory mechanism

Outer ear | Middle ear | Inner ear

Auditory nerve

Air conduction

Bone conduction

FIG. 5-8

Difference in the air and bone conduction pathways in the auditory mechanism.

▼ **Bone conduction** Transmission of sound waves to the inner ear through vibration of the bones of the skull.

become inaudible relatively quickly. When it becomes inaudible, and we place the handle against the mastoid process of the temporal bone just behind our auricle, the tone will be very audible; we are now hearing it by **bone conduction.** We can repeat this exercise and touch the handle (base) of the tuning fork to our chin, our elbow, clavicle, sometimes even our knee, and we will hear the tone by bone conduction propagated across several bones to the cochlea.

We actually hear by bone conduction through three different modes: inertial, compressional, and osseotympanic. **Inertial bone conduction** results from the inertia of the ossicular chain. As the bones of the skull move in vibration, the oval window housing moves as a part of the temporal bone. The inertia of the ossicular chain results in the oval window moving around the stapes; this has the same net effect as the oval window being stationary and the stapes moving, as in air conduction hearing. Inertial bone conduction occurs at all frequencies but is most prominent for lower-frequency sounds.

Compressional bone conduction results from segmental vibration of the bones of the skull. The skull vibrates primarily as a whole at frequencies of about 1500 Hz and lower, but at higher frequencies, different portions may be in different phases. This segmental vibration pattern often results in one portion of the temporal bone moving in one direction and another part moving in the opposite direction, resulting in a compression of the cochlea. The elasticity of the round window membrane and the volume differential between the vestibular and tympanic canals allow for fluid movement, and again, the basilar membrane is stimulated in the same manner as by air conduction. Compressional bone conduction is prominent for frequencies higher than approximately 1500 Hz.

Osseotympanic bone conduction results from the production of air-conducted sound in the external auditory canal by the vibration of the bony walls of the canal. That is, the vibrating bone becomes a source of an air-conducted signal in the external canal. These air-conducted sounds stimulate the tympanic membrane and are transferred through the middle ear to the cochlea. This effect is dramatically enhanced if the canals are plugged so that all the energy in the osseotympanic signal is contained (i.e., none can escape via the external canal). This is called the **occlusion effect**. If we activate a tuning fork (preferably 500 Hz), place the base against our forehead, and plug one ear, we should hear a dramatic increase in loudness in the plugged ear. The occlusion effect is maximal at lower frequencies (i.e., below 1000 Hz).

SIDE NOTES

▼ **Occlusion effect** Production and enhancement of air-conducted sound in a plugged external auditory canal that was originally created by the vibration of the bony walls of the canal.

SUMMARY

Several factors may affect hearing assessment: frequency, duration, and intensity of the auditory stimulus; mode of stimulus presentation (earphones [MAP] or speakers [MAF]); psychophysical methods; and listener characteristics (e.g., preparatory set, age). Hearing sensitivity is dynamic rather than static, and quantification depends somewhat on the definitions used by the examiner.

In clinical assessment of auditory sensitivity and localization of sound sources, the auditory system should be viewed as a part of the total organism. Hearing by bone conduction can be understood better using tuning forks.

The processes discussed here are "normal" in that most of us have them intact, but they clearly are not simple. The role that the auditory system and each of our sensory systems play in our daily lives is extremely complex. This complexity and subtlety of the interaction of our senses can be taken for granted only as long as it functions as intended.

SIDE NOTES

SUGGESTED READINGS

Gelfand SA: *Essentials of audiology,* ed 2, New York, 2001, Thieme.

Martin FN, Clark JG: *Introduction to audiology,* ed 8, Boston, 2003, Allyn & Bacon.

Moore BCJ: *An introduction to the psychology of hearing,* ed 5, San Diego, 2003, Academic Press.

STUDY QUESTIONS

True-False

_____1. The human audibility curve is a graphic representation of auditory sensitivity across frequencies.

_____2. Hearing measured through earphones is more sensitive than hearing measured in a sound field.

_____3. Incident sound is sound reflected from any surface.

_____4. *Azimuth* refers to the location of a sound that is behind the listener.

_____5. The human ear is most sensitive to frequencies between 500 and 4000 Hz.

_____6. A false-positive response occurs when no auditory stimulus is presented.

Fill in the Blank

1. The acoustic effect of a body's presence in a sound field is the _____.

2. The three types of bone conduction are _____, _____, and _____.

3. The head shadow effect is greater for _____ frequencies.

Matching

Match the following terms *(a-g)* with the definitions *(1-7)*.
a. Audiogram
b. Compressional bone conduction
c. Minimum audible pressure
d. Temporal integration function
e. Inertial bone conduction
f. Method of constant stimuli
g. Head shadow effect

1. Change in sensitivity with changes in duration.
2. Auditory sensitivity measured through earphones.
3. Reduction in stimulus intensity at the ear away from the sound source.
4. Graphic representation of threshold for pure tones.
5. Segmental vibration of the bones of the skull.
6. Movement of the oval window relative to the ossicular chain.
7. Two-alternative forced-choice procedure.

MASKING

Masker-Signal Relationships and Sound Level

Masking of Tones by Other Tones
Masking of Tones by Narrow Noise Bands
The Critical Band
Masking of Tones by Wide Noise Bands
Special Cases of Masking

Masking in Clinical Audiology

KEY TERMS

Masking
0 dB effective masking level
Kneepoint
Effective masking
Threshold shift
Upward spread of masking
Narrow-band noise
High-pass filter
Low-pass filter
Band-pass filter
Roll off
Critical band
Wide-band noise
Level per cycle (LPC)
Signal/noise ratio
Simultaneous masking
Forward masking
Backward masking
Masking level difference (MLD)

LEARNING OBJECTIVES

After studying this chapter, the student will be able to do the following:

1. Define masking and explain the importance of quantifying masking in the clinical setting.
2. Describe the concept of the upward spread of masking when pure tones mask other pure tones.
3. Define the concept of 0 dB effective masking level (kneepoint).
4. Identify the concept of critical band and its application to masking.
5. Explain how narrow noise bands mask sound.
6. Identify the three different types of filters and explain how they differ.
7. Define forward masking and backward masking, and describe how they differ.
8. Explain the difference between the concepts of cross-hearing and crossover.
9. Discuss the types of masking used in clinical audiology and the potential problem of cross-hearing.
10. Describe the relationship between masking and bone conduction threshold, and explain how this relationship affects clinical audiometric testing.

▼ **Masking** Process of raising the threshold for one sound by presentation of another sound.

Masking is a process in which the threshold of one sound (signal) is raised by the presentation of another sound (masker). It involves the introduction of a sound to an ear (the *masker*) in order to preclude a person from hearing another sound (the *signal*) in that ear. Masking is quantified as the difference in decibels (dB) between a signal threshold *without* a masker present and the threshold *with* a masker present.

There is no universal classification of the acoustic properties of a masker or a signal. The definition of a "masker" must be made on a case-by-case basis. When we introduce a particular noise to an ear to preclude a person's hearing of a pure tone, clearly the noise is the masker and the pure tone is the signal. However, the situation can be confusing in everyday life, when at one time, for example, a conversation may interfere with (mask) our attention to music, whereas at another time, music may interfere with (mask) our participation in a conversation. This discussion of masking is based on the deliberate introduction of well-controlled sound and well-defined masker-signal relationships.

MASKER-SIGNAL RELATIONSHIPS AND SOUND LEVEL

If we were listening to music with a quiet fan on in the background, the noise of the fan probably would not interfere with our ability to hear the music. However, if the fan noise were progressively increased and the level of the music were held constant, the fan noise would initially be distracting, then the noise would mask the weaker notes in the music, and finally, we would hear only the fan noise, and the music would be inaudible. This phenomenon is even more evident under controlled conditions. If we present a pure-tone signal at threshold, then introduce a noise at a very low level, we may hear both the pure-tone signal and the noise. If we then hold the level of the pure tone constant and progressively increase the level of the noise, eventually the noise level will reach a point that renders the pure tone inaudible.

To make the signal audible in the presence of this noise, we would need to increase the signal level. That is, we have worsened threshold or caused a threshold shift. Each increase in the level of the noise above the point at which the signal becomes inaudible would necessitate an equal increase in the level of the signal to make it audible again. The lowest level of the noise that renders the signal inaudible is referred to as **0 dB effective masking level** or, on a graph, the **kneepoint** (Figure 6-1). Threshold for a signal in the presence of a masker is referred to as the **effective masking** of the masker for that signal.

Masking of Tones by Other Tones

A threshold shift is the numerical difference in dB between a signal threshold in quiet and the threshold obtained with a masker present. The most efficient masker (i.e., provides the most masking for the least amount of energy) for a pure tone is another pure tone of the same frequency. The obvious problem with the use of this type of masker is that the person receiving the signal and masker cannot differentiate the two. However, we can mask one pure tone (the signal) by introduction of another pure tone (masker) of a different frequency. The closer the frequency of the masker is to the frequency of the signal, the more

▼ **Threshold shift** Difference between a stimulus threshold in quiet and in the presence of noise.

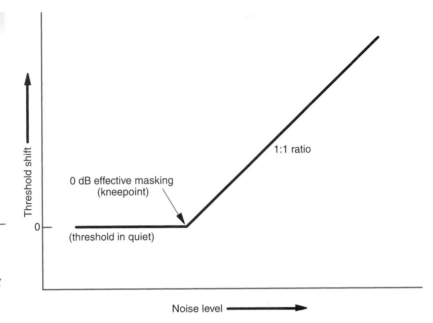

FIG. 6-1

Masking as a function of noise level. (From Deutsch LJ, Richards AM: *Elementary hearing science,* Boston, 1979, Allyn & Bacon.)

efficiently it will mask the signal. However, if the frequencies of the masker and signal are too close, they will not be perceived as different, and then we have the same problem as with using identical masker and signal.

When the level of a masker tone is 60 dB and above, marked differences occur in the masking effects of maskers with frequencies above and below the signal frequency. The masking effect of a tone is much greater *above* the masker frequency than below the masker frequency. Thus, the masking effect spreads rapidly *upward* to higher frequencies (above the masker frequency) as the intensity level of the masker (in dB) is increased, but it extends downward in frequency (below the masker frequency) to only a very limited extent. This is called the **upward spread of masking** (Figure 6-2).

This greater efficiency of a masker to mask higher frequencies may be caused by the shape of the wave envelope on the basilar membrane. Recall that the "tail" of the wave envelope extends toward the base of the cochlea with very little disturbance of the basilar membrane toward the apex from the point of maximum displacement (see Figure 3-8). Further recall that high frequencies maximally displace the basilar membrane toward the base of the cochlea, whereas lower frequencies maximally displace the basilar membrane toward its apex. With these points in mind, we envision the "tail" of the wave envelope of a lower-frequency masker disturbing the basilar membrane in regions receptive to higher frequencies (i.e., toward the base), but not in areas receptive to lower frequencies (i.e., toward the apex).

▼ **Upward spread of masking** Phenomenon in which the masking effect of a tone is greater above the masking frequency than below it.

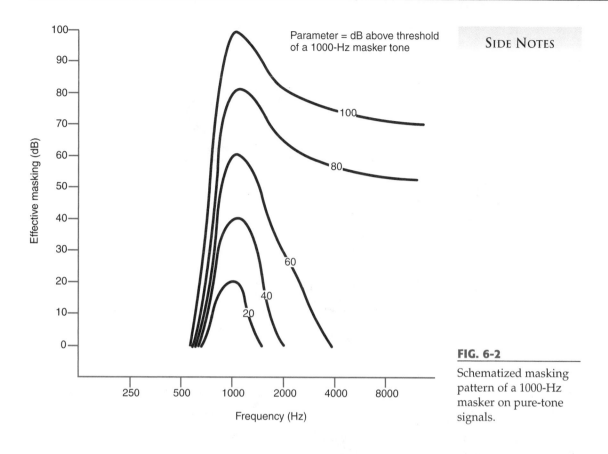

Parameter = dB above threshold
of a 1000-Hz masker tone

y

SIDE NOTES

FIG. 6-2

Schematized masking
pattern of a 1000-Hz
masker on pure-tone
signals.

Masking of Tones by Narrow Noise Bands

Narrow-band noise is noise that is restricted in its frequency range. To produce a narrow-band noise, we employ an electronic filter. The filter allows only the desired frequencies to pass through it. Filters are often classified as high-pass filters (allowing only frequencies above a certain frequency to pass) and low-pass filters (allowing only frequencies below a certain point to pass). Combining high-pass and low-pass filters, we can allow frequencies between two points to pass through; this is called a **band-pass filter.** The frequencies selected as the pass points are called *cutoff frequencies;* that is, they pass frequencies above (high pass) or below (low pass) the selected frequency and reject, or "cut off," frequencies below (high pass) or above (low pass) that frequency. The cutoff normally is not abrupt, but rather progressively attenuates (lessens in value) frequencies more remote from the cutoff frequency. This is called **roll off** and is quantified in dB/octave (Figure 6-3).

▼ **High-pass filter** Electronic filter that allows only frequencies above a certain point to pass through it.

▼ **Low-pass filter** Electronic filter that allows only frequencies below a certain point to pass through it.

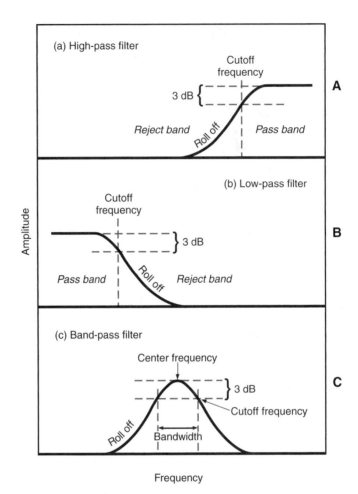

FIG. 6-3

Parameters of three types of filters: **A,** high-pass filter; **B,** low-pass filter; **C,** band-pass filter.

The Critical Band

The use of narrow bands of noise to mask pure-tone signals is based on the critical band concept. It has been determined that only a narrow band of frequencies around the frequency of a given pure tone contributes to the masking of that tone. Frequencies outside this critical band of frequencies add nothing to the masking process.

The concept of critical band in masking is based on the following two primary assumptions:

▼ **Critical band** Range of frequencies around a test frequency that contribute to the masking of that frequency.

- When a tone is masked by noise, only those frequency components in noise that lie in the narrow range around the test frequency are responsible for the masking process. Those frequency components of noise lying outside this "critical band" add nothing to the masking process, but only add to the loudness of the masking noise.

- When a tone is barely masked by noise, the energy content of the noise that falls within the critical band is equal to the energy of the tone.

Narrow-band noise will reach 0 dB effective masking level at a lower sound pressure level (SPL) than white noise. That is, narrow-band noise is a more efficient masker than white noise because it will cause a greater threshold shift than white noise, even though both are of the same intensity (dB SPL) (see later discussion of level per cycle). *Narrow-band noise* consists of noise whose energy content is approximately equally distributed but restricted to a narrow frequency region. On the other hand, *white noise* consists of energy approximately equally distributed over a very wide frequency range. Narrow-band noise is a more efficient masker than white noise because the masking effect of noise on a tone is related only to the energy falling within the critical band of frequencies. Although white noise may have the same overall intensity as narrow-band noise, much of the energy in white noise is not used in the masking process because it falls outside the limits of the critical band.

When a tone is barely masked by noise, energy falling within the critical band of noise equals that of the tone. However, when noise energy falling within the critical band is less than the threshold energy level of the tone being masked, then no threshold shift occurs. The 0 dB effective masking point (kneepoint) of noise is where energy falling within the critical band of noise first equals that of the tone. From this 0 dB effective masking point of noise on, each dB increase in noise energy falling within the critical band will produce an equivalent increase in (worsening of) the pure-tone threshold.

The type of masking employed depends on the auditory stimulus that is intended to be masked. For pure tones, narrow-band noise is the preferred masker. There is a range of frequencies (the *critical band*) surrounding a given stimulus frequency that contribute to the masking of that stimulus. For speech stimuli, a broader band of frequencies is necessary for masking purposes because speech is a broad-band signal. Therefore, wide-band noise, or speech noise (noise designed to duplicate the spectra of speech), is often used as a masker for speech stimuli.

Masking of Tones by Wide Noise Bands

Wide-band noise is an auditory stimulus with equal amplitude of all frequency components. It produces a more generalized masking pattern than narrow bands of noise for broader band stimuli (complex signals). Figure 6-4 represents a wide-band noise with an overall sound pressure level of 80 dB SPL.

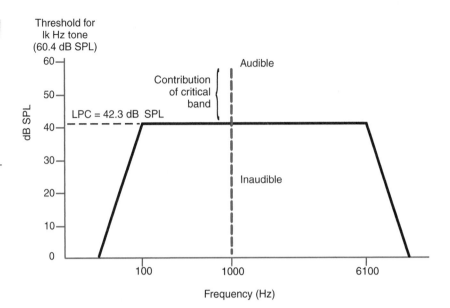

FIG. 6-4

Masking effectiveness of a wide-band noise (overall SPL = 80 dB). Only frequencies in the critical band of the stimulus frequency contribute to the masking. *LPC*, Level per cycle.

Level per cycle (LPC) is the sound pressure level (SPL) of each frequency incorporated into the band of noise. That is, theoretically the band of noise consists of a finite number of pure tones put together in random phase relationships at equal SPLs. The level per cycle of a noise may be estimated by the following simple formula:

$$OASPL - 10(\log_{10} BW) = LPC$$

where *OASPL* is overall sound pressure level of the noise and *BW* is the bandwidth of the noise.

The example in Figure 6-4 is a wide-band noise with a bandwidth of 6000 Hz and an overall sound pressure level of 80 dB SPL. What is the level per cycle?

$$80 - 10 (\log_{10} 6000) = 80 - 10 (3.77) = 80 - 37.7 = 42.3 \text{ dB LPC}$$

That is, our wide-band noise of 80 dB SPL is composed of a large number of pure tones, each at a sound pressure level of 42.3 dB SPL and put together in random phase relationship (see Figure 6-4).

Recall that only a narrow band of frequencies centered around a given pure tone contributes to the masking of that tone (i.e., the critical band). To determine the masking effectiveness of a wide-band noise for a given pure tone, the critical band must be taken into account. This may be accomplished with the following formula:

$$EM = LPC + 10 (\log_{10} CB)$$

where *EM* is effective masking and *CB* is critical band.

The critical band for many pure tones has been empirically determined, and the critical bandwidth is different for each frequency of pure tone. These values may be found in tables in a number of texts.

Q & A

Question:
What is the effective masking (EM) value of a wide-band noise (bandwidth of 6000 Hz) with an overall sound pressure level of 80 dB SPL for a 1000-Hz pure tone?

Answer:
First, we must determine the level per cycle (LPC):

$$LPC = 80 \text{ dB SPL} - 10 \, (\log_{10} 6000)$$
$$= 80 \text{ dB SPL} - 10 \, (3.77)$$
$$= 80 \text{ dB SPL} - 37.7 = 42.3 \text{ dB SPL}$$

Now we apply the formula for effective masking:

$$42.3 \text{ dB SPL} + 10 \, (\log_{10} CB)$$

The critical band for a 1000-Hz pure tone is 64 Hz:

$$\text{Log}_{10} \text{ of } 64 = 1.81$$

Therefore:

$$EM = 42.3 \text{ dB SPL} + 10 \, (1.81) = 42.3 + 18.1 = 60.4 \text{ dB SPL}$$

This means that in the presence of our 80 dB SPL wide-band noise (see Figure 6-4), the threshold for a 1000-Hz tone will be elevated to 60.4 dB SPL. This will vary slightly among individuals because of varying ability to detect a signal in noise, referred to as the **signal/noise ratio.** In testing hearing, we use hearing level (HL) measures. Audiometric zero at 1000 Hz is 7 dB SPL. Therefore, our threshold for a 1000-Hz tone in the presence of this noise will be 53.4 dB HL (60.4 dB SPL – 7 dB SPL).

Special Cases of Masking

Thus far, masking has been discussed in situations in which the masker and maskee are presented together. This is called **simultaneous masking.** However, a masker can provide masking even when it is not actually present at the same time as the signal (maskee). The two conditions in which this phenomenon occurs are when the masker is presented and terminated just before the signal is presented (called **forward masking**) and when the signal is presented and terminated just before the presentation of the masker (called **backward masking**). The time

▼ **Forward masking** Masking of a signal by a masker presented and terminated immediately before the presentation of the signal.

▼ **Backward masking** Masking of a signal by a masker presented immediately after the signal.

separating the masker and maskee must be very brief, with no consistent effect seen in either forward or backward masking when the time separation exceeds 50 msec. The closer in time the signals are, the greater the effect (Figure 6-5).

Another case of masking (or rather "release from masking") may be seen when the relative phases of maskers and signals are manipulated as they are presented binaurally (in both ears). When we present a noise at a comfortable listening level as well as a pulsed tone to the same ear, then adjust the level of the tone until it becomes just inaudible, we have 0 dB effective masking in that ear. This is the standard masking previously discussed. However, if the tone is of low frequency (500 Hz and below), and we add a noise to the other (contralateral) ear, the tone becomes clearly audible in our test ear, even though no changes have been made in the signal or noise in that ear. If we add the same stimulus tone to the other ear, so that each ear now has both stimulus and masker, the stimulus will not be heard in either ear. If we then change the phase of either the signal or the masker by 180 degrees in only one ear, the stimulus will become audible again. This phenomenon is called the **masking level difference (MLD).**

Many combinations of relative phase relationships exist between maskers and signals. Figure 6-6 shows some MLDs along with codes designating the conditions. The MLD is quantified by determining the amount of reduction in masking provided by a particular condition referenced to the condition that provides maximum masking. The condition providing maximum masking is almost always when the signal and masker are presented in phase binaurally (SoNo).

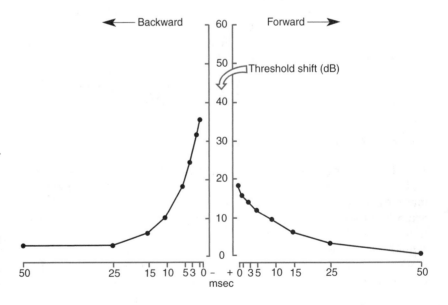

FIG. 6-5

Forward and backward masking in decibels as a function of the interval between signal and masker. (From Elliott LL: *J Acoustic Soc Am*, 34:1108, 1962. Acoustical Society of America.)

Amount of release
from masking

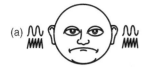

(a) SoNo   0dB   (Signal in phase, noise in phase)

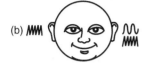

(b) SmNo   9dB   (Signal monaural, noise in phase)

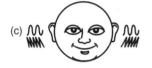

(c) SoNπ   13dB   (Signal in phase, noise 180° out of phase)

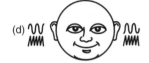

(d) SπNo   15dB   (Signal 180° out of phase, noise in phase)

FIG. 6-6

Masking level
differences (MLDs) for
various conditions.

The MLD is most readily assessed at levels of effective masking of 40 to 50 dB with low-frequency stimuli (200-500 Hz), most often using a wide-band noise as the masker. The greatest effect seen is on the order of 15 dB and is found when comparing the antiphasic (SπNo) condition to the in-phase SoNo condition. The MLD is a fascinating aspect of audition. Simply adding a signal or changing the relative phase of the signal or noise between ears can dramatically change the signal/noise ratio, which underscores the complexity of the central auditory system.

Q & A

Question:
Can the previous information on masking level difference have any practical application?

Answer:
In fact, the MLD has saved many lives. During World War II, pilots and their aircraft were being lost because of their inability to hear and understand communications as a result of aircraft noise. Simply reversing the electrical connections on one earphone (i.e., reversing signal phase) improved this situation considerably. This practical application improved the signal/noise ratio by up to 15 dB by creating the SπNo condition.

MASKING IN CLINICAL AUDIOLOGY

As with other basic psychoacoustic phenomena, masking has important applications in routine clinical audiological practice. Ordinarily, masking is used in clinical audiology when we suspect that a signal presented to an ear being tested (the test ear) is reaching the contralateral ear (the nontest ear) at a level that may be heard in the nontest ear. The principal function of masking noise in audiometry is to eliminate the problem of **cross-hearing,** the unwanted transmission of audible sound from one ear to the other, which may arise under certain conditions for both air and bone conduction measurements (Figure 6-7). If cross-hearing occurs in audiometric testing, the signal intended for one ear would actually be heard by the opposite ear. If unaware of the possibility of cross-hearing, the examiner might erroneously report a threshold on the supposedly tested ear to be lower (better) than it actually is.

▼ **Cross-hearing** Unwanted transmission of audible sound from one ear to the other.

Cross-hearing may occur in air conduction testing whenever there is a relatively large difference between the level of presentation in the test ear and bone-conducted threshold in the nontest ear. The sound presented to the test ear (the stimulus) reaches the nontest ear through bone conduction. The vibration of the earphones and cushion in the test ear sets the bones of the skull into vibration, thereby stimulating the nontest cochlea.

At this point we should distinguish between cross-hearing and crossover. **Crossover** is simply the amount of sound energy that reaches the nontest cochlea through the mechanism previously described. Cross-hearing occurs when crossover exceeds the bone conduction threshold of the nontest cochlea. When testing by air conduction using common

▼ **Crossover** Amount of sound energy that reaches the nontest cochlea by bone conduction.

FIG. 6-7

Effect of cross-hearing on bone- and air-conduction thresholds. If non-test ear (right ear) threshold is 20 dB HL or better, stimulus will be heard and subject will respond.

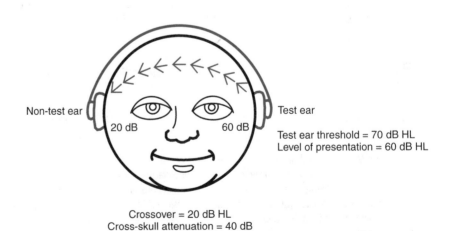

Non-test ear   20 dB   60 dB   Test ear

Test ear threshold = 70 dB HL
Level of presentation = 60 dB HL

Crossover = 20 dB HL
Cross-skull attenuation = 40 dB

audiometric earphones and cushions, crossover is at a level 40 to 60 dB less than the level of presentation in the test ear, whereas crossover is 0 to 10 dB by bone conduction. The difference between the level of presentation in the test ear and crossover to the nontest ear is referred to as **cross-skull attenuation**. In an effort to minimize this problem in clinics, many audiologists use insert earphones that increase the cross-skull attenuation to 90 to 100 dB.

Q & A

Question:
What type of masking is used in clinical audiology?

Answer:
The type of masking used in clinical audiology depends on the nature of the auditory stimulus. For pure tones, narrow-band noise with a bandwidth based on the critical band for each frequency is used. For speech stimuli, we use wide-band noise or spectrally shaped noise called **speech noise** (or **pink noise**).

Interaural attenuation (IA) is insulation provided by the head between the two ears. Clinically, the head provides IA for air-conducted sound of approximately 40 dB. As mentioned, IA can be increased to 90 to 100 dB by using insert earphones. For bone-conducted sound, IA = 0 dB. Thus, the head provides approximately 40 dB of isolation between ears for sounds presented by air conduction, but 0 dB of isolation for bone-conducted auditory stimuli.

The problem of cross-hearing during audiological examination is greatly reduced by masking noise in the better (nontest) ear. This masking elevates the auditory threshold (poorer auditory sensitivity) of the nontest ear so that differences in hearing threshold level (HTL) sensitivity will be reduced. If masking is applied properly and to the proper degree, each ear will be measured in an isolated condition, avoiding cross-hearing. For example, consider a subject in whom the air- and bone-conduction thresholds for the right ear are 0 dB HTL and for the left ear are 60 dB HTL. Cross-hearing might be suspected because of the rather large difference between thresholds of the two ears. To eliminate the possibility of cross-hearing, a masking noise of appropriate intensity is introduced into the better (right) ear and then the auditory sensitivity of the left ear is measured.

Some guesswork is required in masking in clinical audiology because the bone conduction threshold of the nontest ear is not known exactly, and the exact amount of cross-hearing varies from listener to listener. To ensure effective masking, the level of masking applied to the nontest ear must be increased and hearing must be retested three or four times. If the level at which the listener responds to the stimulus in the test ear

SIDE NOTES

▼ **Cross-skull attenuation**
Difference between the level of presentation in the test ear and crossover to the nontest ear.

▼ **Interaural attenuation (IA)** Difference between the level of presentation in the test ear and crossover to the nontest ear.

does not change as the level of masking applied to the nontest ear is increased, we are confident that we have an effective level of masking. However, one caution is necessary here: The masking noise presented to the nontest ear may set the bones of the skull into vibration, just as the auditory stimulus did. This may result in the masking noise crossing over to the test ear, causing overmasking. Fortunately, this phenomenon is not common, generally occurring in patients with severe bilateral conductive hearing loss, and is almost eliminated when insert earphones are used. However, it must be considered.

Q & A

Question:
Why can't we just ask patients/clients to tell us in which ear they hear the stimulus, and thereby know if the stimulus is being heard in the ear being tested?

Answer:
Frequently, patients/clients are not certain in which ear they are hearing the stimulus. At best, this requires a level of sophisticated judgment that is difficult for many listeners to make, particularly hearing-impaired listeners.

SUMMARY

The concept of masking includes the masking of tones by other tones, masking as a function of noise level, the importance of the critical band in masking, wide-band noise as a masker of pure tones, temporal (forward and backward) masking, and masking level difference. Masking in clinical audiology involves the concepts of cross-hearing, cross-skull attenuation, crossover, speech (or pink) noise, and effective masking.

SUGGESTED READINGS

Durant JD, Lovrinic JH: *Bases of hearing science,* ed 3, Philadelphia, 1995, Lippincott Williams & Wilkins.

Martin F, Clark JE: *Introduction to audiology,* ed 9, Boston, 2005, Allyn & Bacon.

Moore BCJ: *An introduction to the psychology of hearing,* ed 5, San Diego, 2003, Academic Press.

Yost WA: *Fundamentals of hearing: an introduction,* ed 5, San Diego, 2006, Academic Press.

STUDY QUESTIONS

True-False

_____1. A high-pass filter blocks sounds below its cutoff frequency.

_____2. Narrow-band noise requires a higher sound pressure level than wide-band noise to reach 0 dB effective masking.

_____3. Masking can occur only when the signal and masker are presented at the same time.

Fill in the Blank

1. The difference between the threshold for a signal in quiet and in the presence of noise is _____.

2. The shape of the wave envelope on the basilar membrane is thought to be responsible for the _____.

3. _____ is used as a masker in clinical audiology for pure-tone testing.

Matching

Match the following terms (a-g) with the definitions (1-7).
a. Forward masking
b. Kneepoint
c. Cross-hearing
d. Masking level difference
e. Crossover
f. Backward masking
g. Masked threshold

1. Masking presented after a signal.
2. Change in phase of stimulus or masker.
3. Masker presented before a signal.
4. Threshold for a signal in the presence of a masker.

5. Sound energy reaching nontest cochlea.
6. 0 dB effective masking.
7. Unwanted transmission of audible sound from one ear to the other that is audible in the non–test ear.

LOUDNESS AND PITCH

7

Loudness

Pitch

KEY TERMS

Equal loudness contours
Phon
Sone
Magnitude estimation
Magnitude production
Sone scale
Ordinal scale
Interval scale
Noy
Loudness
Pitch
Mel scale
Difference tone
Summation tone
Timbre

Side Notes

LEARNING OBJECTIVES

After studying this chapter, the student will be able to do the following:
1. Describe the perceptual concepts of loudness and pitch, and relate them to the physical measurements of intensity and frequency, respectively.
2. Identify the differences between a phon and a sone as units of measurement.
3. Describe ordinal and interval scales and how they differ from each other.
4. Define noy and identify the different variables that can affect noise perception.
5. Explain the mel scale in terms of the relationship of pitch and frequency.
6. Define difference and summation tones, and describe how these phenomena are perceived.
7. Identify how and why timbre is perceived differently from pitch.

Loudness and pitch are the psychological perception of *intensity* and *frequency* of sound, respectively. Intensity and frequency are quantified by means of physical measures of decibels (dB, for intensity) and hertz (Hz, for frequency). However, the quantification of the perception of loudness and pitch is not as straightforward. This chapter addresses the measurement of these subjective perceptions in regard to the objective physical attributes of intensity and frequency.

LOUDNESS

Recall that our auditory sensitivity varies across frequency. The minimum audible pressure (MAP) and minimum audible field (MAF) audibility curves shown in Chapter 5 graphically demonstrate the variation in sensitivity. However, it is not surprising that our perception of loudness also varies across frequency. If we were to present a 1-kHz pure tone at one sound pressure level, then asked listeners to determine a level at which other frequencies of pure tones sound equally loud, and then repeated this process with other sound pressure levels of our 1-kHz tone, the results could be graphically displayed (Figure 7-1).

The curves shown in Figure 7-1 are called **equal loudness contours** and were developed by H. Fletcher and W.N. Munson. Their research

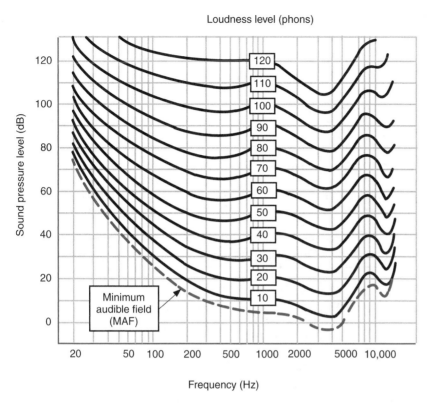

Loudness level (phons)

FIG. 7-1

Equal loudness contours. (Adapted from Robinson DW, Dadson RS: *Br J Appl Phys* 7:166, 1956.)

indicated that at any point along any of the curves, the perceived loudness would be the same. To quantify this relative loudness measure, the unit of measurement developed is called the **phon.** The phon is simply the level in dB of the standard 1-kHz tone against which the subjective loudness of other frequencies is matched. Thus, in Figure 7-1, the 40-dB equal loudness contour is referred to as the 40-phon curve. Any frequency along that curve has a loudness level of 40 phons, regardless of the actual physical measure in dB.

Looking at Figure 7-1, we see that at lower levels, the differences between the physical measurement in dB and the loudness level in phons is very large. At 40 phons, for example, a 1-kHz tone would, by definition, be 40 dB SPL, whereas a 100-Hz tone would be approximately 55 dB SPL, and the two would be judged to be equally loud. At higher levels, the curves flatten somewhat, indicating that the difference in physical magnitude that results in equal subjective perception is less than at lower levels. Looking at the 100-phon curve, a 100-Hz tone would need to be only approximately 105 dB SPL to be equal in loudness level to a 1-kHz tone of 100 dB SPL. The wavelike quality of the curves at higher frequencies most likely represents contributions of canal resonance.

SIDE NOTES

▼ **Phon** Basic measure of loudness; the loudness of a 1000-Hz pure tone at 40 dB SPL is designated as 40 phons.

> ## Q & A
>
> **Question:**
> Does this mean that when we play music through a stereo system at a level lower than it was recorded, there is a perceived loss in fidelity?
>
> **Answer:**
> Yes. Again, looking at Figure 7-1, along the 40-phon contour, the frequencies between 3 kHz and 5 kHz are approximately the same dB SPL, whereas those outside that frequency range vary much more. At very high levels, the phon curves flatten somewhat, so the perceived fidelity may be slightly better. The difficulty is that at these higher levels, the listener may damage his own hearing, and other persons in the area who may not share the desire to hear that music at that time may want to damage the listener! To avoid these difficulties, manufacturers of stereo equipment have developed many electronic compensating mechanisms that differentially amplify the low-frequency and high-frequency ends of the spectra. This works fairly well to compensate for the biological filtering of our auditory systems at lower intensities.

As a unit of measurement, the phon does very well in indicating that two sounds are different in loudness. That is, a sound of 60 phons is definitely louder than a sound of 50 phons. However, the phon measure does not indicate *how much* louder.

S.S. Stevens, a well-known sensory psychologist, developed a loudness scale using a unit of measurement called the **sone.** A physical reference point was arbitrarily selected to be a 1-kHz pure tone at 40 dB SL (sensation level = level above threshold). In a sound field testing environment (see Chapter 5), normal threshold of hearing for trained normal hearing subjects at 1 kHz is approximately 0 dB SPL, so the reference of 40 dB SL is also 40 dB SPL in physical measurement, which is 40 phons on the phon scale and 1 sone on the sone scale. Therefore, the 1-sone reference equates to 40 phons on the phon scale. With this reference established, Stevens had trained listeners either (1) estimate the loudness magnitude of various levels of stimuli presented to them or (2) adjust the level of the stimuli to be twice as loud, half as loud, and so on, relative to the reference 40-phon (1-sone) stimulus. The first technique is called **magnitude estimation,** and the second is called **magnitude production.** The resultant sone scale represents averages obtained from both these techniques. Figure 7-2 represents a comparison of units of measurement of phon and sone.

▼ **Sone scale** Loudness measurement scale in which 1 sone equals 40 phons and 2 sones is twice as loud as 1 sone.

The advantage of the sone scale is that it tells us not only that 2 sones is louder than 1 sone, but also that 2 sones is twice as loud as 1 sone, that 4 sones is twice as loud as 2 sones, and so on. Examination of Figure 7-2 indicates that, for a wide range of sound levels, a change of 10 dB results in a doubling or halving of perceived loudness. Comparing the sone scale to the phon scale, 40 phons is assigned a value of 1 sone, and as a result of findings of the research previously described, we find that

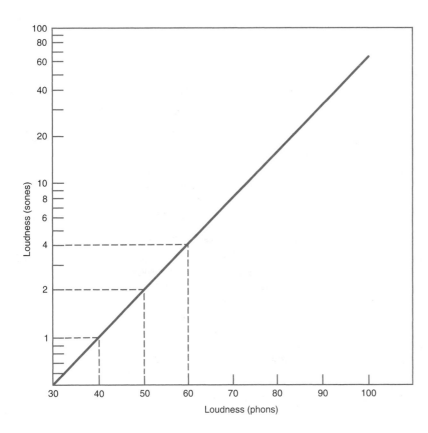

SIDE NOTES

FIG. 7-2

Comparison of phon and sone scales of loudness. (From Stevens SS: *J Acoustic Soc Am* 77:1628, 1985, Acoustical Society of America.)

50 phons is equivalent to 2 sones, 60 phons to 4 sones, 70 phons to 8 sones, 30 phons to 0.5 sones, and so forth.

The *phon* scale is an example of an **ordinal scale**; it shows an order of magnitude (greater than/less than) but makes no attempt to quantify the actual difference in magnitude. On the other hand, the *sone* scale is an example of an **interval scale**; in that we can determine that a sound of 4 sones is half as loud as a sound of 8 sones; the actual difference in magnitude can be specified. Note that the sone scale is considered an interval scale and thus does not include an absolute zero point.

The phon and sone scales, as mentioned, are based on the perception of pure-tone stimuli. For noise-band stimuli, the loudness of a sound at a fixed overall sound pressure level (OASPL) increases when the bandwidth of the noise is expanded to the point that it exceeds the critical band (see Chapter 6). Thus, loudness is not determined only by the sound pressure level (SPL) of the sound but also, to some extent, by the frequency spectrum.

Other perceived qualities of sound, related to but quite different from loudness, are *noisiness* and *annoyance* values. These qualities depend not

▼ **Ordinal scale** Measurement scale that places items in a ranked order, but does not assign intervals between the ranks.

▼ **Interval scale** Scale that assigns items a rank, and on which differences between items may be numerically determined.

only on the SPL but also on spectral distribution, duration, intermittency, and variability of intensity and frequency components in the physical realm. Other factors that can be involved in perceiving sound include predictability, understanding the source of the sound, time of day of occurrence, control of the sound source, and any task involvement of a listener in the psychological realm.

Q & A

Question:
Can we measure the expected perceptual reaction to a sound based on all the variables just listed?

Answer:
We can predict to some extent the reaction to sound, but not nearly as accurately as we can measure loudness. A scale of noisiness includes a unit of measurement called the **noy,** which is based on what we know about the perception of noisiness. The presence of high-frequency components, intermittent presentation versus steady presentation, impulse components, changes in the frequency or intensity of the sound, and higher intensity all add to the perceived noisiness of a sound. The psychological factors are more specific to the situation and the listener. For example, a person working for an airline is less apt to be annoyed by aircraft noise than a person who does not understand or is not interested in the source of the sound. In addition, the person tuning up his motorcycle is apt to enjoy the sound, but his neighbors may not share his enjoyment. Recall that noise has two definitions: the *physical* (being simply aperiodic sound) and the *psychological* (being unwanted sound).

In summary, **loudness** is the subjective perception of the intensity of a sound. It can be measured quite accurately in a controlled environment. The units of measurement of loudness include the phon (which can tell us that one sound is louder than another) and the sone (which can tell us how much louder one sound is than another, for example, twice as loud, four times as loud, and so on). In everyday life, the effect of a given sound depends not only on its loudness but also on many physical and psychological variables.

PITCH

Pitch is the psychological perception of the physical property of frequency. Ordinarily, the higher the frequency of an auditory signal, the higher will be the perceived pitch. However, some sounds do not produce a sensation of pitch. A widely accepted "test" of whether a sound has a perceived pitch is that if it can be used to produce musical melodies, we can be certain that it will produce the sensation of pitch.

Pure tones and most complex sounds do produce the sensation of pitch.

Quantification of the sensation of pitch using pure tones as the signal was undertaken by S.S. Stevens and his colleagues in 1937 and again in 1940. These researchers used two methods in their investigations. One method involved *fractionalization*: a subject was presented with a tone and was asked to adjust the frequency of a second tone until it was perceived as half the pitch of the first tone, one-third the pitch of the first tone, and so on. The second method involved asking subjects to adjust the frequencies of five tones until they were equally different in pitch. That is, they were asked to make the distance in pitch between the first and second tone the same as that between the second and third tone, the third and fourth tone, and so forth. Among the results of these efforts was the development of the **mel scale** of pitch (Figure 7-3).

As with the sone scale, the mel scale is an interval scale that quantifies the difference in pitch; 2000 mels is equivalent to a pitch that is twice that of 1000 mels. On this scale, a 1000-Hz tone at 40 phons of loudness is arbitrarily assigned a value of 1000 mels of pitch. Figure 7-3 shows us that pitch and frequency are not related in a 1:1 ratio. For example, to double the perceived pitch from 1000 to 2000 mels, we must increase frequency from 1000 Hz to approximately 3000 Hz. Figure 7-3 also shows that the audible frequency range of nearly 20,000 Hz is condensed into a pitch range of only approximately 3500 mels. The lowest frequency that typically produces a sensation of pitch is 20 Hz and is assigned a value of zero pitch.

SIDE NOTES

▼ **Mel scale** Psychophysical measure of pitch; the pitch of a 1000-Hz tone at 40 dB SPL is 1000 mels.

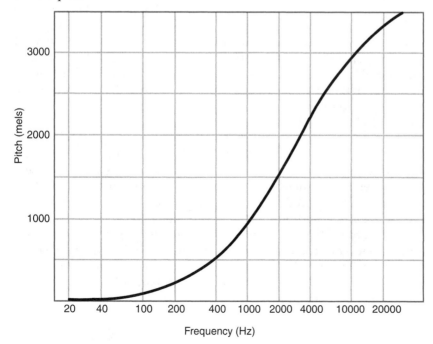

FIG. 7-3
Mel scale, relating frequency to pitch of pure tones.

SIDE NOTES

Q & A

Question:
Does the intensity/loudness of a sound affect its perceived pitch at all?

Answer:
Although there is some disagreement about the magnitude, most researchers have found that generally, low-pitched tones become lower in pitch as intensity is increased, whereas high-pitched tones become higher in perceived pitch as intensity is increased. The division between low-pitched and high-pitched tones is in the area of 500 to 2000 Hz; below and above this range the effect is greatest, whereas within this range there is less effect on the pitch of the tone as intensity is changed.

The pitch of complex sounds appears to be related most closely to the lowest few harmonics of the fundamental frequency (see Chapter 1). If any single harmonic is present at a higher intensity than the remaining harmonics, the higher-intensity harmonic determines the perceived pitch. Pure tones and complex sounds having the same waveform repetition rate may be judged equal in pitch even though their waveform shape is quite different. The relationship between physical and temporal characteristics of sound and the resultant sensation of pitch is not completely understood. Although a detailed discussion of theories of pitch perception is beyond the scope of this text, we present a few phenomena that may provoke some thought and discussion.

If we present a high-frequency tone that is briefly interrupted every 5 msec, the perceived pitch will correspond to that of a 200-Hz tone. Five milliseconds is the period of a 200-Hz pure tone. If the interruptions occur every 10 msec, the perceived pitch will correspond to that of a 100-Hz pure tone, and so on. If we presented tones of 800, 1000, 1200, and 1400 Hz, the listener would perceive a pitch corresponding to 200 Hz, even though no acoustic energy is present at that frequency. The fundamental frequency that would result in harmonics of 800, 1000, 1200, and 1400 Hz is 200 Hz.

▼ **Difference tone** Low-frequency tone perceived by a listener with a frequency that is the difference between two tones presented at a high intensity level, even though no acoustic energy is present at that frequency.

If we present tones of different frequencies at fairly high intensity levels, tones corresponding to the difference in frequency between those tones are often audible even though, again, no acoustic energy is present at the difference frequency. For example, if we presented a 500-Hz tone and a 700-Hz tone simultaneously at 60 dB SPL, the listener would hear a 200-Hz tone in addition to the two primary tones. This is called a **difference tone.** If we presented a 1000-Hz tone and a 500-Hz tone simultaneously at the same intensity, the listener might hear a 1500-Hz tone added. This is called a **summation tone**, which is not as prominent as a difference tone. These are a few of the apparent "mysteries" in the realm of pitch perception.

▼ **Summation tone** High-frequency tone perceived by a listener with a frequency that is the sum of two tones presented at a high intensity level, even though no acoustic energy is present at that frequency.

> **Q & A**
>
> *Question:*
> Do differences in pitch enable us to tell the difference among musical instruments?
>
> *Answer:*
> No. If we heard a musical note such as middle C sounded by a piano, a violin, a trumpet, and a trombone, we would judge them to be the same pitch. The difference that enables us to differentiate the instruments is their difference in quality, which is called **timbre.** Timbre is different from pitch in that it is determined by the whole spectrum that provides the "richness" or "body" of a sound.

SUMMARY

Loudness and pitch are very complex psychophysical phenomena. To some extent, they are each qualitative as well as quantitative phenomena. We can scale both loudness (in phons and sones) and pitch (in mels) with remarkable intrasubject consistency, and yet there are aspects of each that we do not yet fully understand. Neither loudness nor pitch varies directly with its physical counterpart of intensity or frequency, respectively, although each is influenced predominantly by those physical properties.

SUGGESTED READINGS

Gelfand SA: *Hearing: an introduction to psychological and physiological acoustics,* ed 3, New York, 1997, Marcel Dekker, Chapters 11 and 12.

Yost WA: *Fundamentals of hearing: an introduction,* ed 5, San Diego, 2005, Academic Press.

STUDY QUESTIONS

True-False

_____1. A 1-kHz tone at 50 dB SPL has a value of 10 phons.

_____2. The phon scale is an example of an interval scale.

_____3. The loudness of a noise at a fixed overall sound pressure level increases when the bandwidth of the noise exceeds the critical band.

_____4. *Magnitude production* refers to the production of sounds of a given loudness.

_____5. The loudness of a sound does not affect its pitch perception.

Fill in the Blank

1. The phon is a measure of _____.

2. The mel is a measure of _____.

3. *Equal loudness contours* refer to equal perceptions of loudness at different _____.

4. On the phon scale, 40 phons is equal to _____ on the sone scale.

Matching

Match the following terms *(a-e)* with the definitions *(1-5)*.
a. Phon
b. Sone
c. Mel
d. Magnitude estimation
e. Magnitude production

1. Pitch scale
2. Ordinal loudness scale
3. Adjustment of loudness level
4. Judgment of loudness level
5. Interval loudness scale

DIFFERENTIAL SENSITIVITY

The Fechner-Weber Fraction

Difference Limen for Intensity

Difference LImen for Frequency

Temporal Discrimination

KEY TERMS

Just noticeable difference (jnd)
Difference limen
Weber's law (Weber-Fechner law)
Difference limen for intensity (DL_I)
Difference limen for frequency (DL_F)
Difference limen for duration (DL_T)
Temporal resolution
Gap detection threshold

LEARNING OBJECTIVES

After studying this chapter, the student will be able to do the following:
1. Explain the difference between absolute thresholds and difference limens.
2. Identify the three different aspects of differential sensitivity for hearing.
3. Explain how to determine the difference limen for intensity (DL_I).
4. Explain how to determine the difference limen for frequency (DL_F).
5. Explain how to determine the difference limen for time (DL_T).
6. Define gap detection threshold and describe how it is determined.

Differential sensitivity pertains to how much of a change in a physical parameter of a signal must be made before it is noticed by a listener. The minimum change necessary for it to be detected is referred to as a **just noticeable difference (jnd),** or difference limen (*limen* is a German word meaning "threshold").

This chapter discusses a psychophysical principle of the proportional or relative change necessary for detection of a difference, then reviews the research results relating to the jnd for intensity, frequency, and time parameters. Although we are interested here in *sound* as the stimulus and *audition* as the sensory receptor, we will see that general principles of differential sensitivity apply to all sensory input.

THE FECHNER-WEBER FRACTION

Envision carrying an item that weighs 40 pounds. If someone, without our knowledge, carefully adds another item weighing 3 ounces, it is very unlikely that we would notice this added weight. Now picture holding another item weighing only 8 ounces and having the 3-ounce item added again without seeing the addition. In this case we would immediately detect the added weight. Similarly, if we were in a brightly lit room and someone turned on a penlight in a corner of the room, we probably would not notice it. However, if the room was dark or dimly lit, and the same penlight was turned on, we would notice it immediately.

These examples demonstrate that the amount of change in magnitude necessary for the change in weight or light to be noticeable depends on the initial magnitude of the stimulus. That is, the greater the magnitude of the initial stimulus, the greater is the change necessary for a difference to be detectable.

This method of looking at differential sensitivity as a proportional change relative to initial magnitude of a stimulus was formalized by Gustav Fechner and Ernst Weber in the seventeenth century. These scientists developed the following formula:

$$\frac{\Delta I}{I} = k$$

where Δ (delta) indicates change, I is intensity, and k is a constant.

Thus, the formula indicates that the change in stimulus magnitude necessary for it to be detected, divided by the initial magnitude, is a constant. The equation is often referred to as **Weber's law** (or the **Weber-Fechner law**). An example of the application of this principle would be if we held 10 items of equal weight in a basket and could just notice the addition of one more item. Then, if we held 100 of these items in the basket, it would require the addition of 10 more for us to notice the difference.

Q & A

Question:
Does this principle really apply accurately and neatly for all sensory systems?

Answer:
Not quite; research has shown some deviations from Weber's equation in all systems. However, it does give an excellent approximation of changes in stimulus magnitude and perception of those changes.

Detection of small changes in stimulus magnitude is an important aspect of audition for localizing sound sources, appreciating music, and understanding speech. Many auditory cues that we use each day are gained from very small changes in the physical characteristics of sound.

DIFFERENCE LIMEN FOR INTENSITY

The difference limen for intensity may be assessed in a number of ways. One method is to present a *standard tone* that is at some given intensity and ask the subject to judge whether it is of the same or different loudness compared with a second tone of the same frequency that is changed in intensity by the examiner. The minimum physical difference in decibels (dB) necessary to result in a "different" judgment is the difference limen for intensity **(DL$_I$)**.

Another method for assessment of the difference limen for intensity is to present a *steady tone*, then periodically increase its intensity for brief periods. The subject is asked to indicate each time he or she hears this brief increase as the examiner varies the size of the intensity increment. The smallest change in intensity that is detected by the subject is considered his or her DL$_I$.

Another method for determining DL$_I$ is the *beat method*. This method involves simultaneously presenting two tones that are 3 Hz apart in frequency. The beat method results in alternate increases and decreases in intensity as the relative phases change. These are perceived as beats at a rate of three per second when the intensity changes reach the difference limen. This method was employed to obtain the extrapolated data in Figure 8-1. We can see from this figure that both values in dB of ΔI and the $\Delta I/I$ ratio decrease with increasing sensation level (recall that sensation level is dB above threshold).

▼ **Difference limen for intensity** Minimum physical difference in dB necessary to be perceived by a listener.

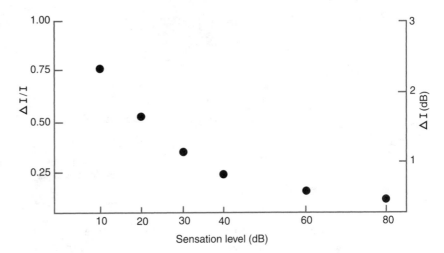

FIG. 8-1
Graph representation of data points taken using the beat method for determining ΔI at various sensation levels of stimulation.

At first glance, Figure 8-1 appears to show a curve that is the opposite of what would be expected based on Weber's law. However, because of the logarithmic method of measuring sound, it requires a progressively larger change in sound pressure to increase sound pressure level (SPL) at higher pressures than it does at low pressures. For example, the change in sound pressure required to increase sound pressure level from 80 to 81 dB SPL is 1000 times greater than that required to increase sound pressure level from 20 to 21 dB SPL (Table 8-1).

This fact at least partially explains why we can detect a 1-dB change in SPL in an 80–dB SPL signal, but usually we cannot detect a 1-dB change in a 20–dB SPL signal. That is, a much greater change in sound pressure is involved in the 1-dB increase from 80 to 81 dB than is involved in the increase from 20 to 21 dB. Thus, the Weber constant applies at least generally to our auditory difference limen for intensity.

TABLE 8-1.   Change in Sound Pressure vs. Change in Sound Pressure Level

Sound Pressure Level (dB SPL)	Sound Pressure (dyne/cm² or Pa)	Difference
Δ from 80 to 81 dB SPL		
80	2.00	
81	2.25	0.25
Δ from 20 to 21 dB SPL		
20	0.002	
21	0.00225	0.00025 (1000-fold increase)

DIFFERENCE LIMEN FOR FREQUENCY

One method for determining the difference limen for frequency involves presentation of a tone of a given frequency and a *comparison tone* that is varied in frequency by the examiner. The subject is asked to judge whether the tones are the same or different. The smallest frequency difference that is judged to be different by the subject is the difference limen for frequency (DL$_F$).

Another approach is to use *frequency-modulated* (FM) *tones* as the stimuli. In this method the test tone frequency is changed, usually at a rate of approximately two times per second, and the subject is asked to indicate when he or she heard the tone "warble." The smallest difference in frequency that produced this perceived warble is the DL$_F$.

Generally, researchers have found that the DL$_F$ becomes smaller as the intensity of the stimuli is increased and becomes larger as the frequency of the stimuli is increased. Data reported from studies of DL$_F$ are not neat, smooth progressions across either frequency or intensity, but often show some aberrant peaks, particularly around 800 Hz. Exactly what causes these irregularities is not known.

▼ **Difference limen for frequency** Smallest difference in frequency that can be detected by a listener.

TEMPORAL DISCRIMINATION

The **difference limen for duration (DL$_T$)** is one of a few measures of temporal discrimination. Assessment of DL$_T$ is most often performed by presenting bands of noise or tones in time intervals indicated by visual cues. The duration of one signal is made longer or shorter than the other (standard), and the subject is asked to report what time interval contained the longer-duration signal. This method is repeated for a range of standard durations, often from 0.1 to 1000 msec, as shown in Figure 8-2. This figure is a "best fit" based on the data of Abel. The smallest difference in duration between the standard and comparison stimuli that results in correct judgments for some predetermined percentage of the time (often 75%) is the DL$_T$.

Another temporal auditory ability is called **temporal resolution.** Several methods are available to assess this ability. Temporal resolution involves the shortest time that is necessary to discriminate between signals. For example, the **gap detection threshold** is a measure of the shortest interruption of a signal, or gap, that can be detected. To determine the gap detection threshold, a tone (or more often a noise) is presented with a very brief interruption (gap) that is varied (Figure 8-3). The subject reports whether he or she detects this gap in the signal as the duration of the gap is shortened.

▼ **Gap detection threshold** Measure of the shortest interruption of a signal that can be detected by a listener.

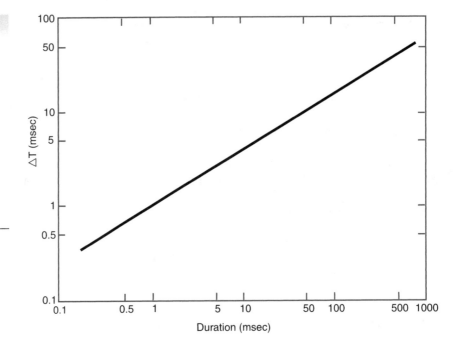

FIG. 8-2

Values of ΔT as a function of duration. (From Abel SM: *J Acoustic Soc Am* 51:1219, 1972, Acoustical Society of America.)

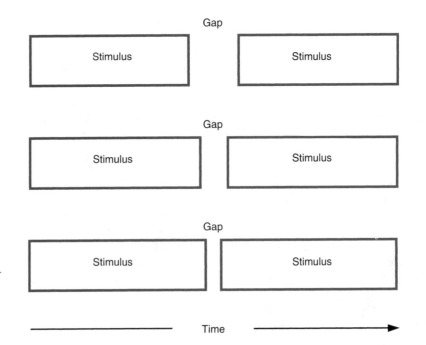

FIG. 8-3

Schematic of gap detection stimuli for three different gap durations.

Many experiments of this type have been conducted, with results indicating that this form of auditory resolution is on the order of 2 to 3 msec. Temporal resolution studies attempt to determine the shortest time necessary for a listener to detect two signals. Using the gap detection threshold method, when the time between signals is shortened beyond the gap detection threshold, the subject hears a steady tone.

SIDE NOTES

SUMMARY

Weber's law is related to differential sensitivity and involves difference thresholds for the parameters of intensity, frequency, and time. This law generally predicts the variations in change of a stimulus necessary to result in detection as the magnitude of standard stimuli is changed. Results vary across subjects, across methods, and across studies. Additionally, some significant differences exist between empirical data and results predicted by Weber's law. However, there is also much agreement. The general principle of magnitude of change necessary for detection increasing with magnitude of the standard stimulus does apply over a wide range of stimulus parameters in all sensory systems.

SUGGESTED READINGS

Moore BCJ: *An introduction to the psychology of hearing,* ed 5, San Diego, 2003, Academic Press.
Yost WA: *Fundamentals of hearing: an introduction,* ed 5, San Diego, 2006, Academic Press.

STUDY QUESTIONS

True-False

_____1. As an auditory stimulus increases in intensity, a greater absolute difference is needed before it can be perceived.

_____2. The difference limen for intensity can be assessed by presenting tones of varying length.

_____3. The gap detection method is a method of assessing temporal summation.

_____4. As the intensity of a stimulus increases, the difference limen for frequency increases.

_____5. As the frequency of a stimulus increases, the difference limen for frequency decreases.

Fill in the Blank

1. Weber's law states that the change in stimulus magnitude necessary for it to be detected divided by the original magnitude is _____.

2. The use of the beat method to determine the difference limen for intensity is based on changes in _____.

Matching

Match the following terms *(a-e)* with the definitions *(1-5)*.
a. Weber's law
b. Beat method
c. Temporal resolution
d. Warble tone
e. Length of two tones judged as the same or different

1. Gap detection threshold.
2. Difference limen for duration.
3. Difference limen for frequency.
4. Difference limen for intensity.
5. Change in stimulus parameter is a constant proportion of initial magnitude of stimulus.

PATHOLOGIES

PATHOLOGIES OF THE AUDITORY MECHANISM

KEY TERMS

Sensory (neural) hearing loss
Central auditory problems
Chondritis
Impacted cerumen
Otitis media
Mastoiditis

Otosclerosis
Ossicular discontinuity
Tinnitus
Temporary threshold shift
Permanent threshold shift
Meniere's disease
Endolymphatic hydrops
Socioacusis
Presbycusis
Cerebrovascular accident
Receptive aphasia

LEARNING OBJECTIVES:

After studying this chapter, the student will be able to do the following:
1. Identify the major pathologies affecting the outer ear, middle ear, and inner ear.
2. Identify congenital problems associated with the central auditory pathways.
3. Describe pathologies affecting the auricle.
4. Define impacted cerumen.
5. Describe pathologies that affect the eustachian tube, the tympanic membrane, and the ossicular chain.
6. Define otosclerosis and discuss how it is surgically corrected.
7. Describe the pathologies of the inner ear that can result from exposure to noise.
8. Identify the complicating factors in detecting and treating noise-induced hearing loss.
9. Recognize the etiologies that can contribute to disorders of the central auditory system.

As seen in Chapter 2, the auditory system can be divided into three major parts: the outer ear, middle ear, and inner ear, as well as the central auditory pathways. Pathologies affecting the outer ear and middle ear are usually medically correctable and produce a type of hearing loss called a *conductive hearing loss* because they cause problems in *conducting* sound energy through the outer ear and middle ear to the inner ear. Pathologies of the inner ear and central pathways, on the other hand, are rarely medically treatable and produce an auditory deficit called a **sensory** (or **neural**) **hearing loss,** or **central auditory problems,** depending on the site of the pathology and the behavioral manifestations.

OUTER EAR PATHOLOGIES

Auricle

The auricle is clearly the most externally exposed portion of the auditory system. Subsequently, many of the pathologies that affect the auricle can incur not only general health problems but cosmetic problems as well. The auricle may be absent *(agenesis)* or deformed *(aplasia)* at birth (Figure 9-1). The extent of these problems varies greatly, from complete absence of all portions of the auricle to a deformation resembling "cauliflower ear."

Chondritis and Cauliflower Ear

The auricle, by virtue of its exposed position, is also susceptible to many acquired disorders. It is often a site of skin disorders, and it may be the only visible portion of the body manifesting signs of a general skin disorder. The auricle may become infected from a person scratching or tugging on it, creating a laceration as an avenue for invasion by bacteria or virus. The auricle may also be affected by environmental effects, such as frostbite. Frostbite may be severe, resulting in a splitting of the skin, which opens an avenue for infection of the underlying cartilage, a condition called **chondritis**.

Repeated trauma to the auricle by any of these means may result in disfiguration referred to as **cauliflower ear** (Figure 9-2). This cosmetic

▼ **Chondritis** Infection of the cartilage.

▼ **Cauliflower ear** Disfiguration of the auricle, resulting primarily from accumulation of blood between the cartilage and its covering.

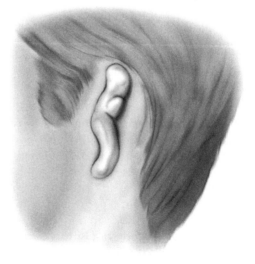

FIG. 9-1

Deformed auricle.

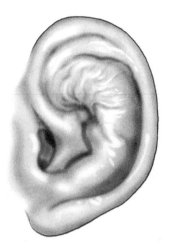

FIG. 9-2

Cauliflower ear.

deformity results primarily from accumulation of blood between the cartilage and its covering. Because of the exposed position of the auricle, it can be readily sunburned. This may be very painful and can also lead to cancers of the skin.

These disorders of the auricle are normally correctable by medical and surgical intervention. It is important that persons with abnormalities of the auricle receive medical attention to prevent the spread of any infectious disorder and to correct cosmetic aspects when desired and feasible.

External Auditory Canal

The external auditory canal may also be affected by congenital (present at birth) disorders. There may be *stenosis* (narrowing of the canal) or congenital *atresia* (complete closure of the canal) (Figure 9-3). Congenital atresia is often accompanied by agenesis of the auricle.

Q & A

Question:
Are congenital problems always limited to the outer ear?

Answer:
These disorders may occur in isolation, or they can be part of several problems resulting from an interruption in fetal development. An interesting finding is that in cases of agenesis of the auricle, if the tragus is present, the cochlea most likely is intact. Conversely, if the tragus is not evident, the cochlea is often affected.

The external auditory canal may also be affected by many viral, fungal, or bacterial infections. One common infection is "swimmer's ear" *(otitis externa)*, caused by heat and moisture associated with swimming, lowering the canal's resistance to infection and creating an environment hospitable to bacteria, fungi, or viruses (Figure 9-4).

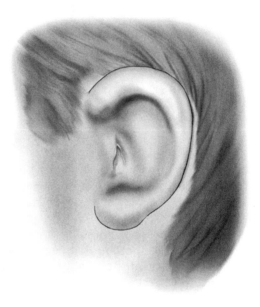

FIG. 9-3

Ear canal atresia.

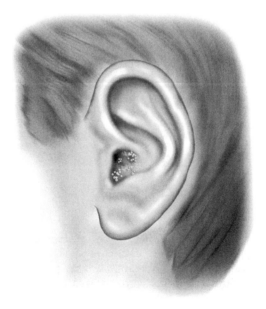

FIG. 9-4

Otitis externa (swimmer's ear).

Impacted Cerumen

Earwax (cerumen) may occlude the canal and become lodged firmly in place. This condition is referred to as impacted cerumen (Figure 9-5). Normally, the outermost layer of skin tissue (epithelium) in the canal migrates from the tympanic membrane, carrying cerumen with it. In addition, cilia (hairs) within the canal also help in moving the cerumen. (In fact, the lining of the external auditory canal and the skin under fingernails and toenails are the only examples of this migratory growth in our bodies.) A damp washcloth moved about the concha and outermost part of the external auditory canal will prevent this cerumen accumulation. It is not necessary to use cotton swabs or other hard, sharp instruments to remove cerumen from the canal, which risks causing great damage and pain.

Sudden head movement with a cotton swab in the canal may result in shoving the tip through the tympanic membrane, possibly into the round window of the cochlea. In the case of a cotton swab penetrating the tympanic membrane only, much pain and often dizziness and nausea can result. In the case of a cotton swab penetrating the round window, a unilateral hearing loss may result in addition to the pain. Furthermore, attempting to remove cerumen with a cotton swab may result in pushing cerumen further into the canal. This may result in impaction of

SIDE NOTES

▼ **Impacted cerumen** Earwax that becomes lodged in the external auditory canal. If enough cerumen accumulates to occlude the canal, a conductive hearing loss will result.

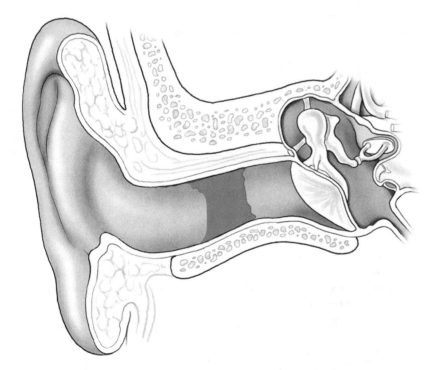

FIG. 9-5

Impacted cerumen (in red).

cerumen and a subsequent conductive hearing loss. Clearly, only the most peripheral areas of the ear should be cleaned in this manner, and it is even worse to clean someone else's ear.

Q & A

Question:
Why do we sometimes cough when something is in our ear?

Answer:
A branch of the cranial nerve X (vagus nerve) that activates the laryngeal area courses very close to the surface of the external auditory canal. Stimulation of this neural path causes the cough reflex. This is another good reason not to "poke around" in the ears.

MIDDLE EAR PATHOLOGIES

Eustachian Tube

The middle ear is a common site for problems to arise. The most common difficulty results from dysfunction of the eustachian tube. Recall that this tube is normally closed at its nasopharyngeal end and opens when we swallow, yawn, or sneeze. Swelling of the tissues near the opening of the tube caused by allergies, trauma, or upper respiratory infection may interfere with normal function.

When the eustachian tube does not open, there is no means of equalizing air pressure between the tympanum and the outside environment. The mucosal lining of the tympanum continues to absorb oxygen and nitrogen from the air, creating a lower air pressure within the tympanum than exists on the outside. This lower pressure results in the tympanic membrane being "pushed" into the middle ear by the relatively higher outside air pressure, thereby increasing the stiffness at the tympanic membrane, which causes some loss of hearing, primarily in the low-frequency range. (*Remember:* An increase in the stiffness component of impedance will provide more opposition to low frequencies.)

This semi-vacuum within the tympanum in some way causes the mucosal lining to begin to secrete a clear fluid. The fluid continues to be secreted as long as the eustachian tube is nonfunctioning. As the fluid accumulates, it exerts an outward pressure against the tympanic membrane. This is normally the stage when a person experiences pain and hearing sensitivity is diminished. If untreated, the pressure of the fluid may increase to the point that it causes the tympanic membrane to burst. At this point, the pain subsides because the fluid is free to drain into the external auditory canal freely with no pressure buildup. The tear in the tympanic membrane may heal, but if the eustachian tube is still not functioning properly, the sequence described will likely be repeated.

Otitis Media

The open communication between the tympanum and the outside environment created by the hole in the tympanic membrane also provides an avenue for infection to invade the middle ear. When this occurs, the condition is called **otitis media** (i.e., infection of the middle ear) (Figure 9-6). This sequence is particularly common in children. The eustachian tube functions optimally when we are in an upright position. Young children spend more time in a prone or supine position and generally have more allergies and upper respiratory infections than most adults, making them more susceptible to eustachian tube dysfunction. In addition, the small size of the eustachian tube in children may cause drainage problems that lead to fluid accumulation and consequent middle ear infections.

Mastoiditis

Otitis media is a potentially dangerous disease of the ear. If otitis media is left untreated, the infection may spread into the air cells of the

SIDE NOTES

▼ **Otitis media** Infection of the middle ear.

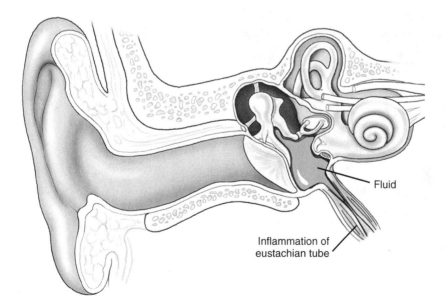

Fluid

Inflammation of eustachian tube

FIG. 9-6

Otitis media.

SIDE NOTES

▼ **Mastoiditis** Infection of the mastoid air cells of the temporal bone.

▼ **Otosclerosis** Abnormal deposits or growths on the stapes, often causing it to be anchored to the oval window and resulting in a conductive hearing loss.

mastoid portion of the temporal bone, a condition known as **mastoiditis**. From here, the infection can also invade the meningeal coverings of the brain after erosion of the tegmen tympani, resulting in *meningitis*.

Therefore, middle ear disorders should be treated by a physician as soon as they are identified. Signs of possible middle ear disease in children include tugging at the ears, unexplained irritability, dark circles under the eyes, persistent upper respiratory difficulty, and drainage from the external auditory canal.

As mentioned, the primary source in the development of this type of middle ear disease is the eustachian tube or, more accurately, some factor (e.g., upper respiratory infection, allergy) that affects eustachian tube function. One medical solution entails surgical implantation of pressure equalization (PE) tubes through the tympanic membrane. These tubes equalize pressure between the tympanum and the outside environment. That is, the tubes perform the job of the eustachian tube on a temporary basis while the cause of tube dysfunction is identified and treated directly. With PE tubes in place, any earache is alleviated and hearing is improved. The patient usually must be careful not to allow water or other possible sources of infection into the external canal while the tubes are in place. However, other than this precaution, children do not seem to be aware of the tubes.

Middle Ear Ossicles

Otosclerosis

Another problem that arises in the middle ear is a disease called **otosclerosis** (Figure 9-7). Otosclerosis is much more common in adults than

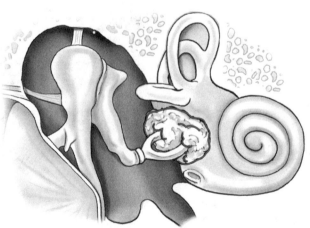

FIG. 9-7

Otosclerosis.

children. The disease consists of abnormal deposits or growth of bone structure, most often around the footplate of the stapes. The bone structure eventually anchors the stapes in the oval window, preventing this ossicle from transferring vibrations to the fluids of the cochlea in the inner ear.

Otosclerosis can be treated surgically by a *stapedectomy*. This procedure involves removal of the stapes and replacement with a prosthesis. The surgery does not take long, with many patients spending no more than one night in the hospital. Stapedectomy has a high success rate and normally completely eliminates the conductive hearing loss caused by otosclerosis. Persons with otosclerosis who choose not to have surgery usually do very well with hearing aids.

Ossicular Discontinuity

Physical trauma can also interfere with middle ear function. Severe blows to the head may affect the middle ear by breaking apart the ossicular chain (called **ossicular discontinuity**), typically at the joint between the incus and stapes (Figure 9-8), or by fracturing the temporal bone. Use of fiber rather than wood or metal seats on swings and laws mandating the use of seat belts in automobiles have reduced this

SIDE NOTES

▼ **Ossicular discontinuity**
Breaking apart of the ossicular chain, usually caused by head trauma, and resulting in a conductive hearing loss.

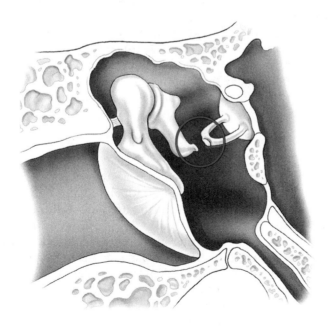

FIG. 9-8

Ossicular discontinuity.

type of middle ear difficulty and other head injuries resulting from a severe blow to the head.

INNER EAR PATHOLOGIES

Cochlea

The cochlea is affected by many factors. Recall that hearing loss resulting from damage to the cochlea rarely responds to medical treatment. The vast majority of persons with sensorineural loss of hearing will have it for the rest of their lives. However, many cases of hearing loss resulting from cochlear damage could have been prevented. Therefore, this section emphasizes what we can do to prevent exposure to the agents that can cause cochlear damage.

Noise

Probably the most common agent that is noxious to the auditory system is *noise*. The hearing loss resulting from exposure to noise is of two types. Most people have been exposed to relatively loud sound and noted later that their hearing was different. They often have a "stuffy" feeling in the ears, a noticeable decrease in hearing sensitivity, and a ringing or buzzing sound in the ears (called **tinnitus**). These symptoms disappear in a day or so, assuming the person does not reenter a noisy environment. This is a noise-induced **temporary threshold shift**.

▼ **Temporary threshold shift** Temporary hearing loss caused by short-term exposure to loud noise.

The second type of hearing loss resulting from exposure to noise is noise-induced **permanent threshold shift**. As the name implies, this hearing loss (and the associated tinnitus) is permanent.

▼ **Permanent threshold shift** Permanent hearing loss caused by continued or repeated exposure to loud noise.

Noise-Induced Hearing Loss

Several factors related to noise-induced hearing loss complicate efforts to prevent it. First, the development is gradual. Initially, only the higher frequencies, usually 3000 to 6000 Hz, are affected, with the individual encountering little noticeable difficulty. With continued exposure to noise, however, the loss of hearing in the higher frequencies worsens, and the range of frequencies affected expands to lower frequencies. The affected person begins to have difficulty understanding speech, particularly in group discussions or when background noise is present. An adult coming into a clinic with noise-induced loss of hearing often states that he or she *hears* well but cannot *understand* the words.

Another perplexing aspect of noise-induced hearing loss is the wide range of individual susceptibility to noise. If a large group of persons were exposed to the same noise over the same period, some would develop extensive hearing loss, whereas others would be minimally affected. At present, no test is available to separate the "tough ears" from the "tender ears."

A third complicating factor, as research has shown, is that noise may produce great physiological damage, primarily destruction of outer hair cells in the cochlea, with little measurable effect on hearing. Whether this damage represents a predisposing or potentiating factor for further damage and greater loss of hearing with continued exposure to noise is not known; however, this would likely affect future hearing loss in some way. Thus, extensive damage to the cochlea may occur long before any resultant loss of hearing can be identified. No test exists for directly assessing damage to the cochlea; assessment of hearing is used to *infer* such damage. Clinical measurement of *otoacoustic emissions,* which are produced by the outer hair cells, has shown promise in detection of this cochlear damage before hearing loss is manifested on an audiogram. In the future, otoacoustic emissions may enable us to identify cochlear damage (outer hair cells) much earlier.

We normally think of noise-induced hearing loss as related to industrial noise. Workers in industrial settings are often exposed to excessive noise and do develop noise-induced hearing loss, despite regulations of the Occupational Safety and Health Administration (OSHA) designed to limit this occupational hazard. Students, particularly those in industrial arts (shop) classes and those participating in shooting sports, are also exposed to high levels of noise. These students are not protected by OSHA regulations and often are not provided with hearing protection. In addition, recreational exposure to noise also takes a toll. Hobbies such as shooting and motor sports, as well as many other activities, are associated with high noise levels. Intelligent use of hearing protection will not reduce the enjoyment of the activity (it may even enhance it), but it will reduce the risk of noise-induced hearing loss.

Noise-induced hearing loss is permanent. The only solution to the problem is prevention. Incorporating good hearing conservation practices and education in industrial arts (shop) and health classes in schools, as well as nonschool hunter education classes, would seem to be a good preventive measure.

SIDE NOTES

Q & A

Question:
If we were to stay in the presence of any noise that causes hearing loss for a long enough time, would we become completely deaf?

Answer:
There is an *asymptotic* level (plateau or upper limit) of threshold shift for any given noise—at least for temporary threshold shift. Evidence also indicates an asymptotic level for permanent threshold shift for any given noise as well. If this is the case, the individual differences seen are in the rate at which people progress toward the asymptotic level, rather than in the ultimate amount of hearing loss developed.

Other Causes of Cochlear Dysfunction

▼ **Meniere's disease** Inner ear disorder that causes fluctuating hearing loss, tinnitus, and vertigo.

Viral infections such as measles and mumps, ototoxic drugs such as streptomycin, and disease processes such as **Meniere's disease** (or **endolymphatic hydrops**) also produce loss of hearing through damage to the cochlea. In these disorders the loss of hearing develops over a short time period. The degree of hearing loss varies greatly, as do the frequencies affected. Public awareness of these diseases and vaccination programs has reduced the prevalence of hearing loss from these factors.

Some sensorineural losses are present at birth (congenital) and may be caused by interruption of fetal development resulting from trauma to the fetus or maternal disorder such as malnutrition or drug ingestion. Other congenital losses may be hereditary, although some hereditary hearing losses do not manifest until well after birth. Identification programs for neonatal hearing loss, which now are mandatory in most states, have aided in early detection of congenital hearing loss. Early detection should result in early habilitation procedures.

Socioacusis and Presbycusis

▼ **Socioacusis (presbycusis)** Loss of hearing associated with aging.

Socioacusis and **presbycusis** each reflect damage to the cochlea. *Presbycusis* is loss of hearing associated with aging. All hearing loss that developed with age was once classified as presbycusis until it was found that the degree of loss that occurred with age varied dramatically in different societies. Following this discovery, the term *socioacusis* was coined to indicate that factors other than aging itself contributed to the deterioration of hearing that occurs with age. The factors thought to influence the magnitude of socioacusis in our society are environmental noise and dietary characteristics. Any exposure to industrial or recreational noise adds to the socioacustic loss of hearing. Although some loss of hearing with age seems to be inevitable, beginning at age 25 to 30 years in our society, prudent use of hearing protection when involved in noisy activities considerably reduces the amount of damage.

CENTRAL AUDITORY SYSTEM DISORDERS

Disorders of the central auditory system are many and varied. Some have shown etiologies (causative factors) such as **cerebrovascular accident** (CVA, stroke) and trauma to the head, which can result in an inability to process language, called **receptive aphasia.** Other cases have no known etiology or lesion, and all we know is that a problem exists. This is often the case with auditory processing disorders. In some cases, such as trauma or CVA, medical intervention is imperative to save a life and to preserve motor, cognitive, and auditory function. In other cases, such as (central) auditory processing disorders, there is no medical treatment.

SUMMARY

This chapter is a cursory review of auditory pathologies. Many texts provide more detail for the interested reader; see the Suggested Readings.

SUGGESTED READINGS

Martin FN, Clark JG: *Introduction to audiology,* ed 9, Boston, 2005, Allyn & Bacon.

Northern JL: *Hearing disorders,* ed 3, Boston, 1996, Allyn & Bacon.

Northern JL, Downs MP: *Hearing in children,* ed 5, Philadelphia, 2002, Lippincott Williams & Wilkins.

STUDY QUESTIONS

True-False

_____1. Conductive hearing losses can usually be corrected by medical or surgical methods.

_____2. Impacted cerumen should never be removed because it protects the tympanic membrane.

_____3. Hearing loss caused by otitis media affects all frequencies equally.

_____4. A temporary threshold shift may be caused by exposure to loud noise.

_____5. Occupational Safety and Health Administration (OSHA) regulations are designed to limit exposure to excessive noise in industrial settings.

_____6. Hearing loss caused by viral infections in the cochlea develops gradually.

Fill in the Blank

1. Deformation of the auricle is usually known as _____.

2. A complication of otitis media is _____.

3. The surgical procedure used to treat otosclerosis is _____.

4. Ototoxic drugs cause damage to the _____.

Matching

Match the following terms *(a-g)* with the definitions *(1-7)*.
a. Receptive aphasia
b. Otitis media
c. Socioacusis
d. Tinnitus
e. Noise-induced hearing loss
f. Agenesis
g. Otosclerosis

1. Permanent threshold shift
2. Abnormal bone growth in middle ear
3. Inability to process language
4. Age-related hearing loss
5. Absence of auricle
6. Ringing or buzzing in ears
7. Eustachian tube dysfunction

GLOSSARY

0 dB effective masking level Lowest level of noise that renders a signal inaudible. Also called *kneepoint.*

10 dB rule Increasing sound pressure level by 10 dB results in a doubling of perceived loudness.

absolute thresholds Lowest limits of auditory awareness.

absolute zero point Nonarbitrary value indicating the absence of the item being measured.

acoustic reflex Contraction of the stapedius muscle in response to external sounds.

air cells Air-filled spaces in the mastoid portion of the temporal bone.

air conduction Transmission of sound waves from the environment through the auricle, the external auditory meatus, and the middle ear to the cochlea in the inner ear.

amplitude Maximum displacement of particles in a medium.

annular ligament Ligament in the middle ear that surrounds the footplate of the stapes to hold it in place.

annulus Ring of fibrous tissue on the outer edge of the tympanic membrane.

ANSI values Guidelines as set by the American National Standards Institute (ANSI).

anterior crus See *crura.*

antihelix Ridge just inside the helix that follows a similar course as the helix.

antitragus Small flap of cartilage that lies just opposite the tragus and forms the inferior boundary of the concha.

aperiodicity Property of a sound wave that is not repeating itself as a function of time. Aperiodic sounds are generally perceived as noise.

areal ratio Difference in the effective areas of the tympanic membrane and the footplate of the stapes. The force is held constant while the area is reduced, resulting in an increase in pressure. Also called *condensation effect.*

attic See *epitympanic recess.*

audiogram Graph or table showing thresholds in hearing level at different frequencies.

auditory branch Portion of cranial nerve VIII coursing from the cochlea to the brainstem.

auditory cortex Areas of the cerebral cortex that are the primary sites for processing auditory information; include the superior gyrus of the temporal lobe and Wernicke's area.

auditory radiations   Multiple small fibers located on the medial geniculate body that transmit auditory stimuli to the auditory areas of the cerebral cortex.

auditory tube   Tube connecting the middle ear cavity to the nasopharynx. Its functions are to equalize pressure in the middle ear, provide an air supply needed for metabolism of the middle ear's tissues, and drain middle ear secretions. Also called *eustachian tube.*

auricle   Outermost portion of the auditory system, forming a cup around the entrance to the external auditory meatus. Also called *pinna.*

azimuth   Angle of incidence of a sound wave as it reaches the head.

backward masking   Masking of a signal by a masker that is presented immediately following the signal.

band-pass filter   Electronic filter that only allows frequencies between two points to pass through it.

bandwidth   Range of frequencies included in a complex sound.

basilar membrane   Tissue that separates the scala media from the scala tympani; holds the organ of Corti.

body baffle   Acoustic effect of the body's presence in the sound field, caused by absorption and reflection of sound by the body.

bone conduction   Transmission of sound waves to the inner ear through vibration of the bones of the skull.

bony labyrinth   See *osseous labyrinth.*

Broca's area   Area on the inferior frontal gyrus of the cerebral cortex; important in the production of speech.

cauliflower ear   Disfiguration of the auricle, resulting primarily from accumulation of blood between the cartilage and its covering.

central auditory system   Subsystem of the human auditory system, consisting of the auditory pathways from the cochlear nucleus to the cerebral cortex.

centrifugal pathway   Descending auditory fibers that descend through the brainstem to the organ of Corti. The system is not well understood but is believed to provide an inhibitory function. Also called *efferent auditory pathway.*

cerebellopontine angle   Junction of the pons and cerebellum; the area of the brainstem that houses the cochlear nucleus and medial opening of the internal auditory meatus.

cerebral cortex   Surface of the brain, consisting of two hemispheres and four lobes in each hemisphere; involved in sensory, motor, and integration functions.

cerebrovascular accident   Abnormal condition of the brain caused by blockage in the blood supply or hemorrhage of a blood vessel in the brain, resulting in death of brain tissue. Depending on the area(s) of the brain involved, speech, language, and auditory abilities may be affected. Also called *CVA* and *stroke.*

cerumen   Waxy lubricant designed to reduce dryness and keep the ear canal supple and clean. Also called *earwax.*

ceruminous glands Glands located in the skin of the cartilaginous portion of the ear canal that produce cerumen (earwax).

characteristic frequency Frequency at which the lowest level of stimulation results in an increase in firing rate.

chorda tympani Branch of the facial nerve that passes through the middle ear and carries information about taste from the anterior portion of the tongue to the central nervous system.

cilia See *stereocilia.*

circular fibers of tympanic membrane Fibers that are arranged in a circular pattern in the tympanic membrane and are sparse near the center and dense toward the periphery.

clinical threshold Lowest sound pressure level to which the subject responds positively at least two of three times during a clinical test.

cochlea Section of the inner ear involved in hearing; contains the organ of Corti, the sense organ for hearing.

cochlear duct See *scala media.*

cochlear microphonic Alternating current (AC) potential in the cochlea that varies in exactly the same manner as the stimulus and is present only while the stimulus is present.

cochlear nerve Branch of cranial nerve VIII that is formed as the hair cells of the organ of Corti synapse with the nerve fibers. Also called the auditory branch of cranial nerve VIII.

cochlear nucleus First major nucleus of the central auditory system, located at the junction of the pons and medulla in the brainstem.

comparison tone Tone varying in small steps around the standard; used for measuring the difference limen.

complex sound Sound that has energy distributed at more than one frequency.

compression Pushing together of particles in a medium, increasing density. Also called *condensation.*

compressional bone conduction Bone conduction resulting from segmental vibration of the bones of the skull. Different portions of the temporal bone vibrate in different phases, resulting in compression of the cochlea.

concha Deepest depression on the auricle, leading directly to and forming the opening to the external auditory meatus.

condensation See *compression.*

condensation effect See *areal ratio.*

conductive hearing loss Hearing loss resulting from impairment to any part of the conductive auditory mechanism.

conductive mechanism Functional component of the auditory system, consisting of the outer and middle ears. Its function is to conduct sound energy from outside the head to be used by the sensory mechanism.

cone of light Reflected spot of light radiating from the center to the periphery of the tympanic membrane when viewed through an otoscope.

contralateral pathway Pathway on the opposite side.

cranial nerve V Trigeminal nerve; innervates the tensor tympani muscle as well as other muscles.

cranial nerve VII Facial nerve; passes through the middle ear superior to the fenestra vestibuli; innervates portions of the face and the stapedius muscle.

cranial nerve VIII Statoacoustic nerve, consisting of auditory and vestibular branches; transmits information about hearing and balance.

critical band Range of frequencies surrounding a given stimulus frequency that contribute to the masking of that frequency. When a tone is just masked by noise, energy falling within the critical band equals that of the tone.

cross-skull attenuation See *interaural attenuation*.

crossed olivocochlear bundle (COCB) See *olivocochlear bundle*.

cross-hearing Unwanted transmission of audible sound from one ear to the other.

crossover Amount of sound energy that reaches the nontest cochlea through bone conduction.

crura Anterior crus and posterior crus; the portions of the stapes that connect its neck to its footplate.

curved-membrane buckling mechanism Greater displacement of the tympanic membrane than of the manubrium of the malleus, resulting in a transfer of force. This results from the edges of the tympanic membrane being firmly attached to the annulus and the inertia of the manubrium.

cutaneous layer of tympanic membrane Outermost layer of tissue comprising the tympanic membrane, continuous with the lining of the external auditory meatus.

cycle Time concept referring to vibrator movement from rest position to maximum displacement in one direction, back to rest, to maximum displacement in the opposite direction, and back to rest again.

damped resonator Resonator that responds to a broad range of frequencies.

damping Rate at which the magnitude of vibration and the loudness of the resultant sound decreases.

decibel Unit of measurement based on logarithms. It is a ratio scale and is applied to the measurement of sound pressure and other variables.

decussate To cross over from one side of the central nervous system to the other.

depolarization Ionic exchange that alters the electrical potential of a hair cell, resulting in the release of a neurotransmitter.

diencephalon Level of the brain just superior to the midbrain.

difference limen (DL) Smallest difference between two stimuli that can be perceived by a listener. Also called *differential threshold* and *just noticeable difference*.

difference limen for duration (DL$_T$) Smallest difference in duration that can be detected by a listener.

difference limen for frequency (DL$_F$) Smallest difference in frequency that can be detected by a listener.

difference limen for intensity (DL$_I$) Smallest difference in intensity that can be detected by a listener.

difference tone   Tone perceived by a listener whose frequency is the difference between two tones presented at a high intensity level, even though no acoustic energy is present at that frequency.

differential threshold   See *difference limen.*

eardrum   See *tympanic membrane.*

effective masking   Threshold for a signal in the presence of a masker.

efferent auditory pathway   See *centrifugal pathway.*

elasticity   Propensity for a medium to return to its original position when the forces of displacement are removed. Also called *springiness* and *stiffness.*

endocochlear potential   Largest of two direct current (DC) potentials that can be measured in the cochlea with no stimulation necessary; seen in the endolymph.

endolymph   Fluid found in the membranous labyrinth.

endolymphatic hydrops   See *Meniere's disease.*

epitympanic recess   Upper region of the middle ear that runs from the upper border of the tympanic membrane to the roof of the middle ear. It contains the head of the malleus and the body and short process of the incus. Also called *attic.*

equal loudness contours   Lines on the phon scale visually representing each phon level. At any point along a single curve, the perceived loudness of that tone would be the same as that of the 1000-Hz tone on that same curve.

eustachian tube   See *auditory tube.*

evoked otoacoustic emissions   Sounds produced by the cochlea in response to stimulation with clicks or carefully selected and arranged pure tones of very brief duration.

expansion   Spreading apart of particles in a medium. Also called *rarefaction.*

external auditory meatus   Canal leading from the auricle to the tympanic membrane; approximately 25-35 mm long, rather narrow, and S shaped. Also called *external auditory canal* and *outer ear canal.*

facial nerve   See *cranial nerve VII.*

false negative   An indicated negative response or lack of response from a subject when a stimulus is detected.

false positive   An indicated positive response from a subject when no stimulus is present or detectable.

fenestra rotunda   Opening in the medial wall of the middle ear cavity inferior to the fenestra vestibuli and covered by a thin, internal tympanic membrane. Also called *round window.*

fenestra vestibuli   Opening in the medial wall of the middle ear cavity that contains the footplate of the stapes. Also called *oval window.*

fibrous layer of tympanic membrane   Middle layer of tissue comprising the tympanic membrane that is primarily responsible for the stiffness of the membrane.

fissure of Sylvius   See *lateral fissure.*

forward making   Masking of a signal by a masker presented and terminated immediately before the presentation of the signal.

Fourier analysis   Mathematical analysis of complex signals into their sinusoidal components.

frequency   Number of complete cycles that occur during a certain period, usually 1 second.

frequency response curve   Graph of the frequencies to which a system will respond and the level of a stimulus necessary for the response to occur. Also called *resonance curve.*

fundamental frequency   Frequency of the lowest component of a complex periodic wave.

gap detection threshold   Measure of the shortest interruption of a signal that can be detected by a listener.

habenula perforata   Tiny openings in the cochlea that allow neural fibers to pass to the organ of Corti.

hair cells   Sensory receptor cells for the hearing process.

harmonic   Component pure tones in a complex periodic signal that are whole-number multiples of the fundamental frequency.

head shadow   Reduction of sound level at the ear farther away from the sound source, caused by the presence of the head between the sound source and the ear. It is a factor in sound localization.

hearing level (HL)   Scale used by audiologists to represent normal human hearing and sensitivity. Also called *hearing threshold level (HTL).*

hearing loss   Inability to perceive the ranges of sound audible to a person with normal hearing.

hearing threshold level (HTL)   See *hearing level.*

helix   Rimlike ridge on the periphery of the auricle. It begins just superior to the opening of the external auditory meatus and runs around much of the periphery of the auricle.

Heschl's gyrus   Gyrus on the medial portion of the temporal lobe running to the superior gyrus of the temporal lobe.

high-pass filter   Electronic filter that allows only frequencies above a certain frequency to pass through it.

human audibility curve   Graphic representation of normal human auditory sensitivity across frequencies.

impacted cerumen   Cerumen that becomes lodged in the external auditory canal and occludes the canal.

impedance   Overall opposition to the flow of energy by a medium; consists of mass, stiffness, and resistance.

incident sound   Sound coming directly from a sound source.

incudomalleolar joint   Articulation between the malleus and the incus.

incudostapedial joint   Articulation between the incus and the stapes.

incus   Middle of the three ossicles that are suspended from the roof of the epitympanic recess; anvil shaped.

inertia   Principle that a body in motion will remain in motion and a body at rest will remain at rest unless acted on by outside forces.

inertial bone conduction   Bone conduction caused by inertia of the ossicular chain. Vibration of the skull causes movement of the oval window while the ossicles' inertia delays their movement.

inferior colliculus   Nucleus in the midbrain where much of the information from the superior olivary complex is received and synthesized, resulting in a localization response.

inner ear   Portion of the auditory and vestibular systems consisting of the cochlea, saccule, utricle, vestibule, and semicircular canals.

inner hair cells   Hair cells that are arranged in one inner row on the organ of Corti. They are pear shaped, and their cilia are arranged in a shallow u pattern.

interaural attenuation   Difference between the level of presentation in the test ear and crossover to the nontest ear. Also called *cross-skull attenuation.*

interaural intensity difference (IID)   Difference in intensity of a sound at the two ears; usually caused by the head shadow effect.

internal auditory meatus   Small channel through the temporal bone that serves as a passage for cranial nerves VII and VIII.

internuncial neuron   Neuron that is innervated by and innervates other neurons within a nucleus.

interval scale   Scale that assigns items a rank and on which differences between items (greater than/less than) may be numerically determined.

ipsilateral pathway   Pathway on the same side.

J.B. Fourier   French mathematician who showed that any complex periodic sound wave disturbance can be mathematically broken down into sine waves that vary in terms of frequency, amplitude, and phase relations.

just noticeable difference   See *difference limen.*

kneepoint   See *0 dB effective masking level.*

labyrinth   Mazelike, interconnecting, fluid-filled canals that form the inner ear.

labyrinthine wall   Medial wall of the middle ear that separates it from the inner ear.

lateral fissure   Fissure separating the temporal lobe from the frontal and parietal lobes of the brain. Also called *fissure of Sylvius.*

lateral lemniscus   Primary afferent central auditory tract connecting the superior olivary complex to the inferior colliculus.

lateralization   Effect of detecting a sound with a greater intensity in one ear relative to the other ear as being located nearer to the ear receiving the more intense stimulus. If the sound intensity changes in one ear, the listener will perceive the sound source as moving.

lenticular process   Portion of the incus that articulates directly with the head of the stapes.

level per cycle   Sound pressure level of each frequency incorporated into a band of noise.

lever action   Lever formed by the manubrium of the malleus and the long process of the incus, resulting in a reduction of movement from the malleus to the incus and a consequent increase in force/unit area across the ossicular chain.

lobule   Most inferior landmark on the auricle, composed of soft tissue and highly vascular in nature. Also called *lobe.*

logarithm   A form of mathematical notation based on exponents.

longitudinal fissure   Space that separates the two hemispheres of the cerebral cortex.

loudness   Subjective perception of intensity.

low-pass filter   Electronic filter that allows only frequencies below a certain frequency to pass through it.

MAF   See *minimum audible field.*

magnitude estimation   Estimation of loudness magnitude of various levels of stimuli relative to a standard.

magnitude production   Production of sounds to match or relate to a standard stimulus.

malleus   Most lateral of the three ossicles that are suspended from the roof of the epitympanic recess; hammer shaped.

manubrium   Portion of the malleus that connects directly to the tympanic membrane and is visible upon otoscopic examination of the ear.

MAP   See *minimum audible pressure.*

maskee   Sound that cannot be detected because of the presentation of another sound.

masker   Sound that raises the threshold of another sound.

masking   Process of raising the threshold for one sound by the presence of another sound.

masking level difference (MLD)   Phenomenon in which a signal may be made audible in the presence of masking noise by changing the relative phase of the signal or masker.

mass   Any form of matter (solid, liquid, or gas). Also, one energy-storing component of impedance. Opposes high frequencies maximally.

mass-stiffness gradient   Difference in width and thickness (i.e., relative mass and stiffness) from the base to the apex of the basilar membrane. It results in variations in resonance at different locations of the basilar membrane.

mastoid air cells   Air-filled spaces in the mastoid portion of the temporal bone.

mastoid portion of temporal bone   Portion of each temporal bone that is behind the auricle, containing numerous air-filled spaces called *air cells.*

mastoiditis   Infection of the mastoid air cells of the temporal bone.

medial geniculate body   Nucleus located in the thalamus that is the starting point for auditory radiations, which run to the auditory cortex.

mel scale   Psychophysical scale of pitch that relates the pitch to frequency of pure tones.

membranous labyrinth   Part of the labyrinth inside the bony labyrinth that is composed of soft tissue and consists of a series of communicating sacs and ducts that conform to the shape of the larger bony labyrinth. It is filled with endolymph.

Meniere's disease   Inner ear disorder that causes fluctuating hearing loss, tinnitus, and vertigo. Also called *endolymphatic hydrops.*

method of adjustment Method of testing auditory sensitivity in which the subject adjusts some parameter of the stimulus, usually the intensity level.

method of constant stimuli Method of testing auditory sensitivity by using a two-alternative forced-choice procedure. After an approximation of sensitivity is obtained using another method, several levels above and below the approximation are selected and presented in random order.

method of limits Method of testing auditory sensitivity in which the examiner changes a parameter of the auditory stimulus and the subject indicates when the stimulus is detected.

middle ear Hollow, air-filled cavity located medial to the tympanic membrane between the outer ear and the inner ear. It is located within the temporal bone and is where airborne sound is converted to mechanical energy.

middle ear transformer Combined factors of areal ratio, the lever action of the malleus and incus, and the curved-membrane buckling mechanism of the tympanic membrane that serve as an impedance-matching mechanism between the outside air and the dense fluid of the inner ear.

minimum audible angle Smallest separation of angles of incidence that can be perceived.

minimum audible field (MAF) Lowest level of sound heard when stimuli are presented through speakers.

minimum audible pressure (MAP) Lowest level of sound heard when measuring auditory sensitivity through earphones.

molecule Microscopic particle that makes up matter.

narrow-band noise Noise that is restricted in its frequency range.

nasopharynx Uppermost portion of the pharynx (throat).

natural frequency See *resonant frequency.*

noise Sound that lacks cyclical or repetitive (periodic) vibrations (physical), or unwanted sound (psychological).

noise-induced hearing loss See *permanent threshold shift.*

nominal scale Measurement scale that places items into categories, but does not order them.

normal hearing 0 db hearing level; the median thresholds for many young adults with no auditory pathology. This is the reference used for testing in a clinical setting.

noy Measure of noisiness.

nucleus of lateral lemniscus Area of synapses within the lateral lemniscus.

occlusion effect Production and enhancement of air-conducted sound in a plugged external auditory canal that was originally created through the vibration of the bony walls of the canal.

olivocochlear bundle (OCB) Portion of the descending efferent auditory system, descending from the superior olivary complex to the organ of Corti. The two components are the *crossed olivocochlear bundle (COCB)*, which stimulates the contralateral cochlea, and the *uncrossed olivocochlear bundle (UOCB)*, which stimulates the ipsilateral cochlea.

ordinal scale Measurement scale that places items in a ranked order, but does not assign intervals between the ranks.

organ of Corti   Sensory end organ of hearing.

oscillation   Back-and-forth motion, such as that of a pendulum.

osteotympanic bone conduction   Bone conduction resulting from the production of air-conducted sound in the external auditory canal caused by vibration of the bony walls of the canal.

osseous labyrinth   Outer portion of the labyrinth that is filled with perilymph and surrounds the membranous labyrinth. It contains the cochlea, the three semicircular canals, and the vestibule. Also called *bony labyrinth.*

ossicles   Three small bones—the malleus, incus, and stapes—that cross the middle ear cavity and transmit vibrations from the tympanic membrane to the inner ear mechanism. Also called *ossicular chain.*

ossicular discontinuity   Breaking apart of the ossicular chain, usually caused by head trauma and resulting in a conductive hearing loss.

ostium   Opening to a body cavity; specifically, the nasopharyngeal opening of the eustachian tube.

otitis externa   See *swimmer's ear.*

otitis media   Infection of the middle ear.

otoacoustic emissions   Sounds produced by the cochlea. They may be evoked or spontaneous.

otosclerosis   Abnormal deposits or growths on the ossicles, often causing the stapes to be anchored to the oval window and resulting in conductive hearing loss.

otoscope   Instrument used to examine the external auditory meatus and the tympanic membrane. It consists of a light, a magnifying lens, and a speculum.

outer ear   Outermost portion of the auditory system, consisting of the auricle (pinna) and external auditory meatus.

outer ear canal   See *external auditory meatus.*

outer hair cells   Hair cells that are arranged in three or four outer rows on the organ of Corti. They are cylindrical in shape, and their cilia are arranged in a w pattern.

oval window   See *fenestra vestibuli.*

pars flaccida   Small, triangular area on the superior portion of the tympanic membrane that contains few fibers and is flaccid in nature. Also called *Shrapnell's membrane.*

pars tensa   Largest portion of the tympanic membrane, containing numerous fibers that contribute to the taut nature of the membrane.

particle displacement   Distance that particles are displaced from their rest positions.

peak amplitude   Linear measurement of a wave from the baseline to the point of maximum displacement.

peak-to-peak amplitude   Linear measurement of a wave from the point of maximum displacement in one direction to the point of maximum displacement in the other direction.

perichondritis   Infection of the cartilage. Also called *chondritis.*

perilymph   Fluid found in the osseous labyrinth of the inner ear.

period   Time needed for a vibrator to complete one complete cycle of vibration; the reciprocal of frequency.

periodicity   Property of a sound wave repeating itself as a function of time.

peripheral auditory system   Anatomical subsystem of the human auditory system, consisting of the outer, middle, and inner ears.

permanent threshold shift   Permanent hearing loss caused by continued or repeated exposure to loud noise. Also called *noise-induced hearing loss.*

petrous portion of temporal bone   Portion of each temporal bone that is located at the base of the skull and contains the essential parts of the organs of hearing and equilibrium.

phase   Point in the cycle at which a vibrator is located at a given instant in time.

phon scale   Basic measurement scale of loudness. The loudness of a 1000-Hz pure tone at 40 dB SPL is designated as 40 phons.

physicists' zero   Basic reference for all sound pressure measurement; 20 µPa (twenty micropascals). It is the smallest pressure variation from ambient pressure produced by a 1-kHz pure tone that could be detected by young listeners with no auditory pathology and who were trained in detection of this signal.

pink noise   See *speech noise.*

pinna   See *auricle.*

pitch   Subjective perception of frequency.

posterior crus   See *crura.*

preparatory set   Subject's predisposition to respond to a stimulus; can be altered by the examiner's instructions.

presbycusis   Hearing loss resulting from the aging process.

pressure equalization (PE) tubes   Tubes surgically implanted in the tympanic membrane that serve to equalize middle ear air pressure in cases of eustachian tube dysfunction.

promontory   Projection on the medial wall of the middle ear inferior to the fenestra rotunda that is created by protrusion of the first turn of the cochlea.

psychophysical method   A means of coupling physical properties of a stimulus to the perception of and response to that stimulus. Various psychophysical methods are used to assess auditory sensitivity.

psychophysical scale   Scale that attempts to quantify a relationship of a subjective sensation and a physical quantity.

pure tone   Sound that has almost all its energy located at one frequency. It is the basic component of all sound.

pyramidal eminence   Prominence on the posterior side of the middle ear cavity that contains the stapedius muscle.

radial fibers of tympanic membrane   Fibers that originate near the center of the tympanic membrane and spread toward the periphery.

rarefaction   See *expansion*.

ratio scale   Measurement scale having all properties of nominal, ordinal, and interval scales as well as possessing true zero points, such that exact ratios between items may be determined. It is the most precise scale type.

receptive aphasia   Inability to process language.

reflected sound   Sound that is reflected from any surface.

Reissner's membrane   Tissue that separates the scala vestibuli from the scala media.

resistance   Dissipation of energy, occurring primarily by conversion to heat; the energy-dissipating component of impedance; has equal effect at all frequencies.

resonance   Increase of overall amplitude of vibration caused by a similar or identical periodic energy source being activated.

resonance curve   See *frequency response curve*.

resonant frequency   Frequency at which a system will most easily be set into vibration. It is the point at which the effects of mass and stiffness are equal.

response pattern   Firing-rate variations of a neuron in response to stimulation.

rest position   Point of origin of a particle (i.e., with no external forces operating).

reverberation   Multiple or continuous reflections of sound that prolong the existence of the sound within a confined space.

roll off   Rate of progressive attenuation from a cutoff frequency of a filter, quantified in dB per octave.

root mean square (rms)   Mathematical measurement of amplitude of sound pressure; the square root of the average of all instantaneous variations of pressure squared within the sine wave. In a sinusoid, it is equivalent to 0.707 times the peak value.

round window   See *fenestra rotunda*.

saccule   One of two communicating sacs found in the membranous labyrinth. Along with the utricle, it plays a role in maintaining spatial orientation.

scala media   Middle of the three canals within the cochlea; contains the organ of Corti. Also called *cochlear duct*.

scala tympani   One of the three canals within the cochlea, separated from the scala media by the basilar membrane.

scala vestibuli   One of the three canals within the cochlea, separated from the scala media by Reissner's membrane.

scaphoid fossa   Depression on the auricle between the helix and antihelix.

sebaceous glands   Oil-producing glands located in the skin of the cartilaginous portion of the ear canal. They produce an oily component of earwax (cerumen) to keep the ear canal supple and reduce dryness.

Second-order neuron   Second neuron in a sensory pathway; many have complex response patterns. In the auditory system, the neurons that synapse with cranial nerve VIII fibers in the cochlear nucleus are second-order neurons.

semicircular canals   Three canals, each of which represents a body plane in space and moves in conjunction with head and body activity; provide information to the brain about head position and movement.

sensation level   Decibel (dB) scale in which the listener's threshold is the zero point; the number of dB above a listener's threshold.

sensory hearing loss   Hearing loss caused by pathology of the inner ear, usually not medically treatable.

sensory mechanism   Functional component of the auditory system, consisting of the inner ear.

Shrapnell's membrane   See *pars flaccida.*

signal   Sound to which a listener attends.

simple harmonic motion   See *sinusoidal motion.*

simultaneous masking   Presentation of the masker and maskee at the same time.

sine wave   Temporal picture of cyclical variations. Also called *sine curve.*

sinusoidal motion   Disturbance in a medium in which particles are displaced perpendicular to the direction of the disturbance. Also called *simple harmonic motion.*

socioacusis   Loss of hearing associated with aging and societal factors noxious to the auditory system, such as noise and dietary factors.

sone scale   Loudness measurement in which 1 sone is equal to 40 phons and 2 sones is twice as loud as 1 sone, 4 sones is twice as loud as 2 sones, etc.

sound   Condition of disturbance of particles in a medium.

sound field testing   Presentation of auditory stimuli for testing through speakers.

sound pressure level (SPL)   Scale that measures amplitudes in terms of dynes/cm^2 or pascals (Pa). The reference point for this scale is 0.0002 dyne/cm^2, or 20 μPa, and the measurement is expressed in decibels (dB).

sounding board resonance   Tendency of an object to vibrate most vigorously when it comes in contact with a sound source closest to its resonant frequency. The increased size of the vibrating surface leads to an increase in sound level. Similar to *sounding board effect.*

spectral envelope   Graphic representation of the distribution of energy across frequency for a complex sound.

spectrum   Graph that displays amplitude across frequency.

speech noise   Noise designed to duplicate the speech spectrum, used as a masker for speech stimuli in clinical audiology. Also called *pink noise.*

spiral limbus   Point of attachment for the tectorial membrane within the organ of Corti.

spontaneous otoacoustic emissions   Otoacoustic emissions that are produced without stimulation.

spring-mass model   Visual model that shows the properties of molecular elasticity.

springiness   See *elasticity.*

squamous portion of temporal bone   Portion of each temporal bone that contributes to the lateral wall of the cranium and contains the opening of the external auditory meatus.

standard tone   Tone used as a reference to compare the parameters of other tones.

stapedectomy   Surgical procedure consisting of removal of the stapes and replacement with a prosthesis; performed to restore hearing in patients with otosclerosis.

stapedius muscle   One of two middle ear muscles; the smallest striated muscle in the human body, located in the posterior portion of the middle ear cavity. It connects to the neck of the stapes and, on contraction, causes an increase in stiffness of the ossicular chain.

stapes   Most medial of the three ossicles that are suspended from the roof of the epitympanic recess; stirrup shaped.

statoacoustic nerve   See *cranial nerve VIII.*

stereocilia   Small, hairlike projections on the tops of the inner and outer hair cells. Each outer hair cell has as many as 150 stereocilia, and each inner hair cell has 50 to 70 stereocilia. Displacement of the stereocilia results in depolarization and neural discharge. Also called *cilia.*

stiffness   See *elasticity.*

stria vascularis   Vascular complex that maintains the chemical composition of the endolymph in the cochlea.

summating potential   Stimulus-related direct current (DC) response in the cochlea.

summation tone   Tone perceived by a listener whose frequency is the sum of two tones presented at high intensity levels, even though no acoustic energy is present at that frequency.

superior gyrus   Uppermost gyrus of the temporal lobe of the cerebral cortex.

superior olivary complex   Major nucleus in the medulla. It receives input from both ears, and its primary function is to code information used in the localization of sound.

swimmer's ear   Infection in the external auditory canal. It may be viral, fungal, or bacterial and often results from heat and moisture in the canal. Also called *otitis externa.*

tectorial membrane   Structure sitting above the organ of Corti and attached at the spiral limbus. It is in contact with the stereocilia of the outer hair cells, causing movement of the stereocilia when the basilar membrane is displaced.

temporal bone   Paired cranial bone of the skull that houses the middle and inner ear structures. It consists of four parts: the squamous portion, the mastoid portion, the petrous portion, and the tympanic portion.

temporal integration   Change in threshold as the duration of a stimulus changes. Also called *temporal summation.*

temporal resolution   Ability to distinguish two sounds and interpret them as separate sounds.

temporal summation   See *temporal integration.*

temporary threshold shift   Temporary hearing loss caused by short-term exposure to loud noise.

tensor tympani muscle   One of two middle ear muscles, located in the anterior portion of the middle ear cavity. It is connected to the manubrium of the malleus and, on contraction, moves the malleus medially and anteriorly, thus stiffening the middle ear mechanism.

thalamus   Major distribution center for sensory and motor activity, located in the diencephalon.

threshold   Minimum intensity at which a stimulus can be detected.

threshold shift   Numerical difference between the threshold before and the threshold during or after exposure to an agent that affects threshold.

timbre   Quality of a tone determined by the whole spectrum that provides the "richness" or "body" of a sound.

tinnitus   Ringing or buzzing sound in the ear.

tip links   Links on inner hair cells that run from the body of stereocilia to the tip of adjacent stereocilia. The links stretch when the basilar membrane is displaced.

tracking threshold   Method of recording a subject's response stimulus over time and across frequencies, in which the subject controls the stimulus intensity and is asked to keep the signal barely audible.

tragus   Small flap of cartilage on the anterior wall of the external auditory meatus.

transduction   Change in the form of energy.

trapezoid body   Neural tract that crosses the brainstem at the level of the superior olivary complex. Approximately two thirds of the nerve fibers cross to the contralateral side.

traveling wave   Complex pattern of vibration of the basilar membrane as pure-tone disturbances grow in magnitude from the base to the resonant point on the basilar membrane.

triangular fossa   Depression on the auricle medial to the scaphoid fossa in the superior portion of the auricle between the helix and antihelix.

trigeminal nerve   See *cranial nerve V.*

tuning curve   Record of the responsiveness of a single hair cell to a variety of frequencies.

two-alternative forced-choice procedure   Psychophysical test measuring the limits of a client's threshold by presenting sound levels in a random order and asking the client to indicate whether or not the auditory stimulus was present in a given time period.

tympanic cavity proper   Main portion of the tympanic cavity. It lies between the tympanic membrane and the inner ear and contains the ossicles. Also called *tympanum.*

tympanic membrane   Elastic structure that separates the outer ear from the middle ear cavity. Also called *eardrum.*

tympanic portion of temporal bone   Portion of each temporal bone that forms sections of the external auditory meatus.

tympanic sulcus   Groove in the bony wall of the external auditory meatus that holds the annulus of the tympanic membrane.

tympanum   See *tympanic cavity proper.*

umbo   Center point of the tympanic membrane, representing the projection from the manubrium of the malleus.

uncrossed olivocochlear bundle (UOCB)   See *olivocochlear bundle.*

undamped resonator   Resonator that responds to a narrow range of frequencies.

upward spread of masking   Phenomenon in which the masking effect of a tone is greater above the masking frequency than below it.

utricle   One of two communicating sacs found in the membranous labyrinth. Along with the saccule, it plays a role in maintaining spatial orientation.

velocity   Speed of sound through a transmitting medium.

vestibular nerve   Branch of cranial nerve VIII that originates from the vestibular portion of the inner ear and joins with the cochlear nerve.

vestibular portion   Section of the inner ear that is concerned with the sense of balance and spatial orientation.

vestibule   Central part of the labyrinth.

waveform   Graph that displays variations in pressure in relation to amplitude and time.

wavelength   Distance a wave disturbance travels during one complete cycle of vibration.

Weber's constant   Formula $\Delta I/I = k$, where I represents intensity, Δ indicates change, and k is a constant. Also called *Weber's fraction.*

Weber's law   Law stating that a stimulus must be changed by a constant proportion of itself to be judged as different. It is represented by the formula $\Delta I/I = k$. Also called *Fechner-Weber law.*

Wernicke's area   Area of the left temporal lobe of the cerebral cortex that is important in the comprehension of speech.

white noise   Wide-band stimulus with equal energy at each frequency within its spectrum.

Whole-nerve action potential   Response that originates in cranial nerve VIII (CN VIII). It is seen only at the onset of an abrupt signal and represents the synchronous discharge of many CN VIII nerve fibers.

wide-band noise   Wide-band auditory stimulus with equal amplitude at each frequency component.

zero-dB hearing level   The zero reference used in clinical testing. It is the median threshold for young adults with no auditory pathology and varies by frequency. Zero reference is established by the American National Standards Institute (ANSI).

zero-degree azimuth   Orientation of a sound source directly in front of the listener.

CHAPTER STUDY QUESTIONS AND ANSWERS

CHAPTER 1 STUDY QUESTIONS

True-False

_____1. Hertz (Hz) is a measurement of wavelength.

_____2. White noise has energy distributed evenly throughout the sound spectrum.

_____3. The decibel scale is a linear scale.

_____4. A medium that returns to its original shape is said to possess elasticity.

_____5. Resistance causes a vibrating body to remain in motion.

_____6. For resonance to occur in a tube, the tube length must be half the wavelength of the resonant frequency.

Fill in the Blank

1. A sound that has almost all its energy located at a single frequency is a _____.

2. A wave shape that does not repeat itself as a function of time is a _____ sound disturbance.

3. The process of changing energy from one form to another is _____.

4. When testing hearing, audiologists use the _____ scale.

5. A graph showing amplitude as a function of frequency is called a _____.

Matching

a. Amplitude
b. Impedance
c. Reverberation
d. Decibel
e. Sound
f. Pitch
g. Inertia

_____1. A condition of disturbance of particles in a medium.

_____2. A body in motion remains in motion.

_____3. Maximum displacement of particles in a medium.

_____4. The perceptual correlate of frequency.

_____5. Unit of measurement of amplitude of a signal.

_____6. Repeated reflection of sound.

_____7. Opposition to flow of energy.

CHAPTER 2 STUDY QUESTIONS

True-False

_____1. The stapedius muscle is attached by means of a tendon to the neck of the stapes.

_____2. The conductive mechanism of the human auditory system resides primarily in the outer ear.

_____3. Damage to the outer ear or middle ear is permanent and not medically treatable.

_____4. The middle ear is an impedance-matching mechanism.

_____5. The footplate of the stapes rests in the fenestra rotunda (round window).

_____6. The tympanic membrane consists of three layers of tissue.

_____7. The acoustic reflex is a startle response.

Fill in the Blank

1. The innermost (medial) ossicle in the middle ear is the _____.

2. The orifice of the auditory (eustachian) tube that opens when we swallow, yawn, or sneeze is located in the _____.

3. The instrument used to view the external auditory meatus and tympanic membrane is the _____.

Matching

a. Annulus
b. Tympanum
c. Condensation effect (areal ratio)
d. Auditory (eustachian) tube
e. Cranial nerve VII (facial nerve)
f. Lever ratio
g. Cranial nerve V (trigeminal nerve)

_____1. The tympanic membrane is approximately 17 times as large in area as the footplate of the stapes.

_____2. The manubrium of the malleus is approximately 1.3 times the length of the long process of the incus.

_____3. A connective tissue ring that retains the perimeter of the tympanic membrane.

_____4. Innervation of the stapedius muscle.

_____5. Middle ear cavity.

_____6. Pressure equalization function.

_____7. Innervation of the tensor tympani muscle.

Anatomy Labeling

1. Landmarks of the auricle

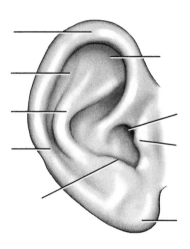

2. Basic anatomy of the ear: outer, middle, and inner ear

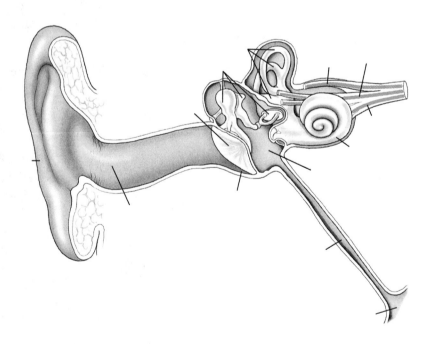

3. Tympanic membrane

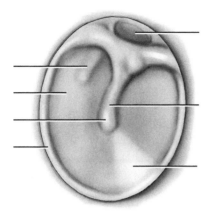

4. Middle ear

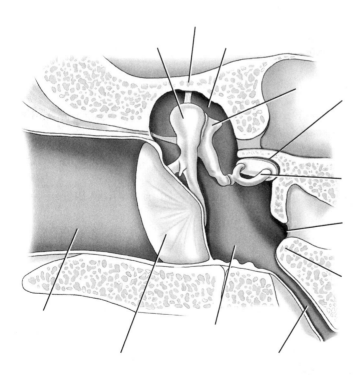

5. Ossicles

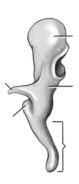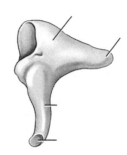

CHAPTER 3 STUDY QUESTIONS

True-False

_____1. The bony labyrinth is filled with endolymph.

_____2. The cochlea is divided into three canals.

_____3. The basilar membrane separates the scala tympani from the scala vestibuli.

_____4. Inner hair cells contain fewer cilia than outer hair cells.

_____5. The organ of Corti receives nutrients from the stria vascularis.

_____6. The basilar membrane is wide and thick at the apex and narrow and thin at the base.

Fill in the Blank

1. The fluid-filled canals of the inner ear are called the _____.

2. The _____ contains the footplate of the stapes.

3. The two branches of cranial nerve VIII are the _____ and _____ branches.

4. The pattern of vibration of the basilar membrane is best described as a _____.

Matching

a. Hair cells
b. Tuning curve
c. Otoacoustic emissions
d. Stria vascularis
e. Habenula perforata
f. Perilymph
g. Organ of Corti

_____1. Sensory end organ of hearing.

_____2. Sensory receptors for hearing.

_____3. Openings in the cochlea for inner radial fibers of cranial nerve VIII.

_____4. Blood supply to the cochlea.

_____5. Fluid found in the osseous labyrinth.

_____6. Responsiveness of a neuron to a variety of frequencies.

_____7. Sounds produced by the cochlea.

Anatomy Labeling

1. Bony labyrinth

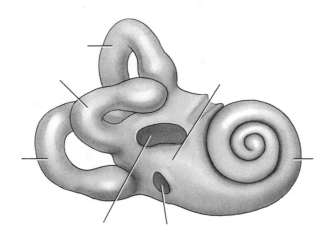

2. Membranous labyrinth

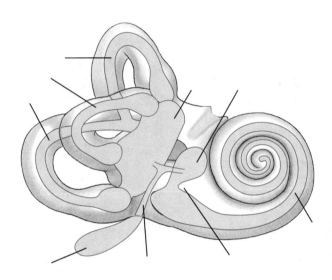

3. Cochlea

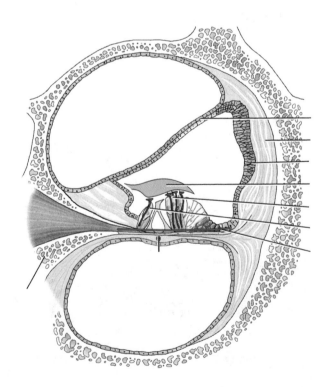

4. Organ of Corti cross section

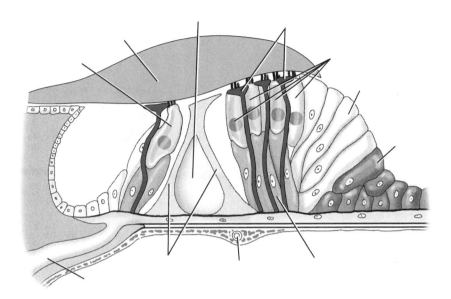

5. Branches of cranial nerve VIII

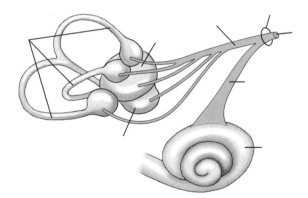

CHAPTER 4 STUDY QUESTIONS

True-False

_____1.   The first major nucleus in the central auditory system is the trapezoid body.

_____2.   Fibers can cross from one side of the central nervous system to the other at the cochlear nucleus.

_____3.   Most afferent cranial nerve VIII primary fibers are innervated by inner hair cells.

_____4.   Perception of loudness and pitch takes place within the auditory cortex.

_____5.   The localization response begins in the inferior colliculus.

Fill in the Blank

1.   The first point in the central auditory system to receive input from both cochleas is the _____.

2.   The _____ connect the medial geniculate body to the auditory cortex.

3.   The medulla, pons, and midbrain are all parts of the _____.

4.   Neurons that connect other neurons to each other are called _____ neurons.

Matching

a.   Speech reception
b.   Medulla
c.   Speech production
d.   Thalamus
e.   Efferent auditory pathway
f.   Midbrain

_____1.   Medial geniculate body

_____2.   Wernicke's area

_____3. Superior olivary complex

_____4. Inferior colliculus

_____5. Broca's area

_____6. Olivocochlear bundle

Anatomy Labeling

1. Lateral view of the brain

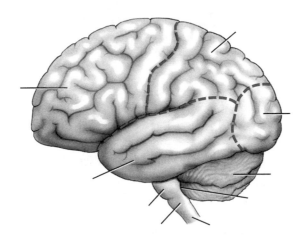

2. Midsagittal view of the brain

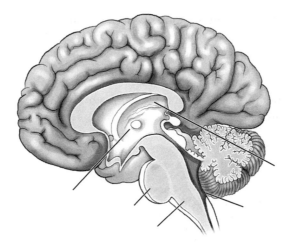

3. Superior view of the brain

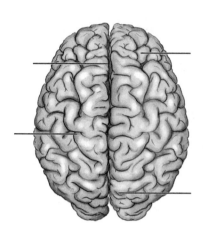

CHAPTER 5 STUDY QUESTIONS

True-False

_____1. The human audibility curve is a graphic representation of auditory sensitivity across frequencies.

_____2. Hearing measured through earphones is more sensitive than hearing measured in a sound field.

_____3. Incident sound is sound reflected from any surface.

_____4. *Azimuth* refers to the location of a sound that is behind the listener.

_____5. The human ear is most sensitive to frequencies between 500 and 4000 Hz.

_____6. A false-positive response occurs when no auditory stimulus is presented.

Fill in the Blank

1. The acoustic effect of a body's presence in a sound field is the
   _____.

2. The three types of bone conduction are _____,
   _____, and _____.

3. The head shadow effect is greater for _____ frequencies.

Matching

a. Audiogram
b. Compressional bone conduction
c. Minimum audible pressure
d. Temporal integration function
e. Inertial bone conduction
f. Method of constant stimuli
g. Head shadow effect

_____1. Change in sensitivity with changes in duration.

_____2. Auditory sensitivity measured through earphones.

_____3. Reduction in stimulus intensity at the ear away from the
           sound source.

_____4. Graphic representation of threshold for pure tones.

_____5. Segmental vibration of the bones of the skull.

_____6. Movement of the oval window relative to the ossicular chain.

_____7. Two-alternative forced-choice procedure.

CHAPTER 6 STUDY QUESTIONS

True-False

_____1. A high-pass filter blocks sounds below its cutoff frequency.

_____2. Narrow-band noise requires a higher sound pressure level than wide-band noise to reach 0 dB effective masking.

_____3. Masking can occur only when the signal and masker are presented at the same time.

Fill in the Blank

1. The difference between the threshold for a signal in quiet and in the presence of noise is a(n) _____.

2. The shape of the wave envelope on the basilar membrane is thought to be responsible for the _____.

3. _____ is used as a masker in clinical audiology for pure-tone testing.

Matching

a. Forward masking
b. Kneepoint
c. Cross-hearing
d. Masking level difference
e. Crossover
f. Backward masking
g. Effective masking

_____1. Masking presented after a signal.

_____2. Change in phase of stimulus or masker.

_____3. Masker presented before a signal.

_____4. Threshold for a signal in the presence of a masker.

_____5. Sound energy reaching nontest cochlea.

_____6. 0 dB effective masking.

_____7. Unwanted transmission of audible sound from one ear to the other that is audible in the non–test ear.

CHAPTER 7 STUDY QUESTIONS

True-False

_____1. A 1-kHz tone at 50 dB SPL has a value of 10 phons.

_____2. The phon scale is an example of an interval scale.

_____3. The loudness of a noise at a fixed overall sound pressure level increases when the bandwidth of the noise exceeds the critical band.

_____4. *Magnitude production* refers to the production of sounds of a given loudness.

_____5. The loudness of a sound does not affect its pitch perception.

Fill in the Blank

1. The phon is a measure of _____.

2. The mel is a measure of _____.

3. *Equal loudness contours* refer to equal perceptions of loudness at different _____.

4. On the phon scale, 40 phons is equal to _____ on the sone scale.

Matching

a. Phon
b. Sone
c. Mel
d. Magnitude estimation
e. Magnitude production

_____1. Pitch scale

_____2. Ordinal loudness scale

_____3. Adjustment of loudness level

_____4. Judgment of loudness level

_____5. Interval loudness scale

CHAPTER 8 STUDY QUESTIONS

True-False

_____1. As an auditory stimulus increases in intensity, a greater absolute difference is needed before it can be perceived.

_____2. The difference limen for intensity can be assessed by presenting tones of varying length.

_____3. The gap detection method is a method of assessing temporal summation.

_____4. As the intensity of a stimulus increases, the difference limen for frequency increases.

_____5. As the frequency of a stimulus increases, the difference limen for frequency decreases.

Fill in the Blank

1. Weber's law states that the change in stimulus magnitude necessary for it to be detected divided by the original magnitude is _____.

2. The use of the beat method to determine the difference limen for intensity is based on changes in _____.

Matching

a. Weber's law
b. Beat method
c. Temporal resolution
d. Warble tone
e. Length of two tones judged as the same or different

_____1.   Gap detection threshold.

_____2.   Difference limen for duration.

_____3.   Difference limen for frequency.

_____4.   Difference limen for intensity.

_____5.   Change in stimulus parameter is a constant proportion of initial magnitude of stimulus.

CHAPTER 9 STUDY QUESTIONS

True-False

_____1.   Conductive hearing losses can usually be corrected by medical or surgical methods.

_____2.   Impacted cerumen should never be removed because it protects the tympanic membrane.

_____3.   Hearing loss caused by otitis media affects all frequencies equally.

_____4.   A temporary threshold shift may be caused by exposure to loud noise.

_____5.   Occupational Safety and Health Administration (OSHA) regulations are designed to limit exposure to excessive noise in industrial settings.

_____6.   Hearing loss caused by viral infections in the cochlea develops gradually.

Fill in the Blank

1. Deformation of the auricle is usually known as _____.

2. A complication of otitis media is _____.

3. The surgical procedure used to treat otosclerosis is _____.

4. Ototoxic drugs cause damage to the _____.

Matching

a. Receptive aphasia
b. Otitis media
c. Socioacusis
d. Tinnitus
e. Noise-induced hearing loss
f. Agenesis
g. Otosclerosis

_____1. Permanent threshold shift

_____2. Abnormal bone growth in middle ear

_____3. Inability to process language

_____4. Age-related hearing loss

_____5. Absence of auricle

_____6. Ringing or buzzing in ears

_____7. Eustachian tube dysfunction

CHAPTER 1 ANSWERS

True-False

1. F (frequency)
2. T
3. F (ratio)
4. T
5. F (inertia)
6. F (one quarter)

Fill in the Blank

1. pure tone
2. aperiodic
3. transduction
4. hearing level
5. spectrum

Matching

1. e
2. g
3. a
4. f
5. d
6. c
7. b

CHAPTER 2 ANSWERS

True-False

1. T
2. F (middle)
3. F (it is normally treatable)
4. T
5. F (oval window)
6. T
7. F (occurs at lower levels than needed for startle)

Fill in the Blank

1. stapes
2. nasopharynx
3. otoscope

Matching

1. c
2. f
3. a
4. e
5. b
6. d
7. g

Anatomy Labeling

1. Landmarks of the auricle—refer to Figure 2-3.
2. Basic anatomy of the ear: outer, middle, and inner ear—refer to Figure 2-4.
3. Tympanic membrane—refer to Figure 2-5.
4. Middle ear—refer to Figure 2-8.
5. Ossicles—refer to Figure 2-13.

CHAPTER 3 ANSWERS

True-False

1. F (perilymph)
2. T
3. F (scala tympani from scala media)
4. T
5. F (spiral arteries)
6. F (reverse)

Fill in the Blank

1. labyrinth
2. fenestra vestibuli (oval window)
3. auditory, vestibular
4. traveling wave

Matching

1. g
2. a
3. e
4. d
5. f
6. b
7. c

Anatomy Labeling

1. Bony labyrinth—refer to Figure 3-1.
2. Membranous labyrinth—refer to Figure 3-2.
3. Cochlea—refer to Figure 3-3.
4. Organ of Corti cross section—refer to Figure 3-4.
5. Branches of cranial nerve VIII—refer to Figure 3-5.

CHAPTER 4 ANSWERS

True-False

1. F (cochlear nucleus)
2. F (superior olivary complex)
3. T
4. F (occurs at lower centers)
5. T

Fill in the Blank

1. superior olivary complex
2. auditory radiations
3. brainstem
4. internuncial

Matching

1. d
2. a
3. b
4. f
5. c
6. e

Anatomy Labeling

1. Lateral view of the brain—refer to Figure 4-2, *A*.
2. Midsagittal view of the brain—refer to Figure 4-2, *B*.
3. Superior view of the brain—refer to Figure 4-2, *C*.

CHAPTER 5 ANSWERS

True-False

1. T
2. F (reverse)
3. F (directly from noise)
4. F (any angle)
5. T
6. T

Fill in the Blank

1. body baffle effect
2. inertial, compressional, osteotympanic
3. higher

Matching

1. d
2. c
3. g
4. a
5. b
6. e
7. f

CHAPTER 6 ANSWERS

True-False

1. T
2. F (reverse)
3. F (reminder: forward and backward masking)

Fill in the Blank

1. threshold shift
2. upward spread of masking
3. Narrow-band noise

Matching

1. f
2. d
3. a
4. g
5. e
6. b
7. c

CHAPTER 7 ANSWERS

True-False

1. F (50 phons)
2. F (ordinal)
3. T
4. T
5. F (loudness can affect pitch)

Fill in the Blank

1. loudness
2. pitch
3. frequencies
4. 1 sone

Matching

1. c
2. a
3. e
4. d
5. b

CHAPTER 8 ANSWERS

True-False

1. T
2. F (intensity)
3. F (temporal resolution)
4. T
5. F (increases)

Fill in the Blank

1. constant
2. relative phase

Matching

1. c
2. e
3. d
4. b
5. a

CHAPTER 9 ANSWERS

True-False

1. T
2. F (should be removed when it occludes canal)
3. F (primarily low frequencies)
4. T
5. T
6. F (often causes sudden hearing loss)

Fill in the Blank

1. cauliflower ear
2. mastoiditis
3. stapedectomy
4. cochlea

Matching

1. e
2. g
3. a
4. c
5. f
6. d
7. b

INDEX

Page numbers followed by "f" indicate figure.